The
Peanut Ball

Penny
Thank you for all
your support over the
years and for training me all
those years ago! Thanks for giving
me encouragment to make this dream
come true to get peanut balls in
L&D all over the world. See page 13
as I am so grateful for your
mentorship and the world to
take this to the world. I
was glad to see you in
Houston.
Hugs and Love
Cheri

The Peanut Ball

BASIC AND ADVANCED TECHNIQUES

for Use During Labor and Delivery

Cheri Grant, RN

"The Peanut Ball Lady"

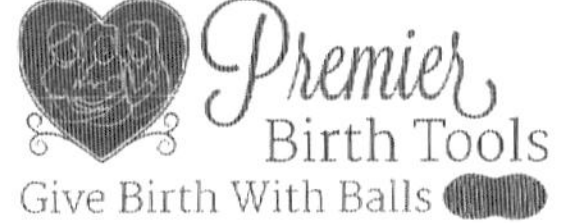

The Peanut Ball: Basic and Advanced Techniques for Use During Labor and Delivery

Requests for information should be addressed to:

Premier Birth Tools LLC
premierbirthtools@gmail.com
P.O Box 294
Owasso, Oklahoma 74055

ISBN 978-0-9971782-0-3

Cover design by lindseybeharry.com
Edited by Susan Troy

Printed in the United States of America

To my daughters, Crystal and Tiffany,
for their love and support to create this book,
and showing me the joy of birth.

To all the couples who have let me
share in their birth experiences and help
create special birth memories.

To the doulas, nurses, and midwives everywhere,
who assist their clients during childbirth.

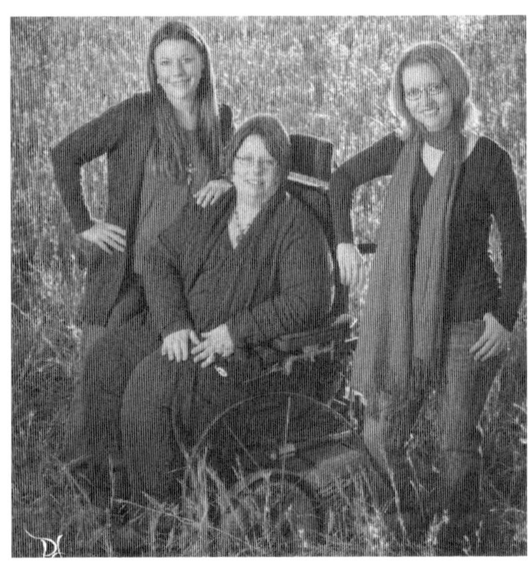

Crystal, Cheri, and Tiffany

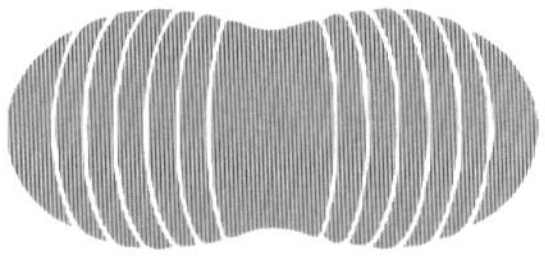

CONTENTS

ACKNOWLEDGMENTS

I WOULD LIKE TO THANK Penny Simkin, my mentor, for her inspiration and reassurance, and Susan Troy for her commitment and support in making my dream come true.

A special thanks to doulas, nurses, and mothers who have supported this book through pictures, demonstration, and assisting in research projects.

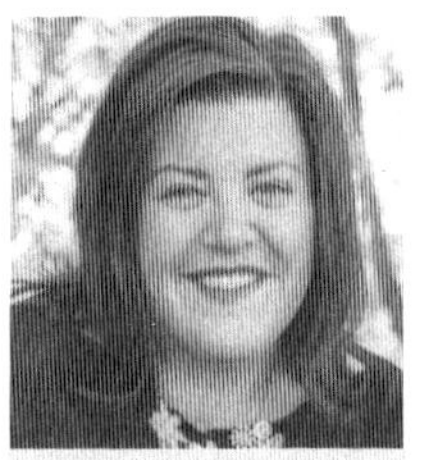

Editor and friend, Susan Troy

Mothers: Brittni Jernigan, Nicole Biggs, Bethany Hanrieder, Lilly Seng, Debbie Pienta and other mothers. Doulas: Hillary Goodner, Marlita Camacho, Janell Cornelius, Toni Nolan, Kimmie Stratmann, Tess Hartsell, Natalia Helmerich. Missy David, Sarah Coffin, Hannah Lawrence, Kasy Wixon, Diane Daniel, and Danielle Lugrand.

Peanut Ball Ambassadors: Rebekah Porter, Tammy Ryan, and future and all other Peanut Ball Ambassadors mentioned in the book.

Photographers: Chelsea Evans Photography, Samantha Steen Photography, and Tamera Edwards Photography.

Peanut Ball Trainers: Heather Turner, Melissa Harley, Heidi Duncan, Mandy Irby, Amy Emerson, Amy Bookwalter, Megan Honaker, Emma Whitlock, Marques Scott, Stephanie Assouline, Megan Honaker, Nona Barnett, Amy Wilt, Kelby Propp, Brandi Patrick, and future Peanut Ball Trainers.

Midwives: Gail Tully, Ruth Cobb, and Regina Kizer.

Nurses: Lynn Clutter, Sarah Lavonne, Bethany Hanrieder, Heather

Knife-Chief, Nikki Zerfas, Polly Perez, Julie Broaddrick, Jennifer Reimer, Amy Rice, Bonnie Craig, Krista Gosnell, April Coulter, and Becky Cartwright. This book would not have been possible without each one of you.

FOREWORD

HEATHER S. TURNER, CD (DONA), LCCE

Authorized Peanut Ball Trainer
"Your Birth" navydoula.com

I FIRST MET CHERI in 2014 at the LAMAZE/DONA conference in Kansas City, Missouri. She invested her time and patience to explain all the outstanding benefits of using the peanut ball during Labor and Delivery. The next morning, I attended her standing-room-only session "The Peanut Ball: New Tool for your Doula Bag and Its Effect on Laboring Women" and was blown away.

Since then, her extensive knowledge and research on the use of peanut balls and their benefits, combined with her ability to convey the information to the birthing community, has proven invaluable. Most inspiring is her goal of a peanut ball in every Labor and Delivery room.

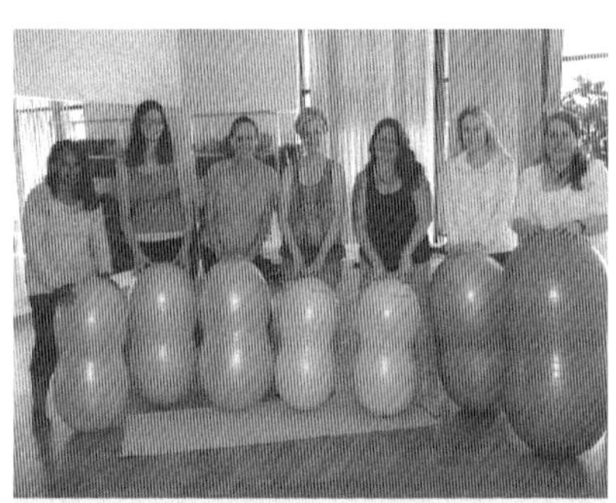

Heather Turner with "Your Birth" Authorized Peanut Ball Trainer Workshop

I am thrilled to be Premier Birth Tools' first Authorized Peanut Ball Trainer and I am honored that Cheri has grown to be a wonderful friend and caring mentor. Congratulations on your new book; I have no doubt you will continue to amaze our birthing community!

Cheri, congratulations on a wonderful accomplishment! This book will delight the Labor and Delivery nurse and give practical relief for the birthing parents of many new generations to come

Gail Tully, CPM, Spinning Babies®

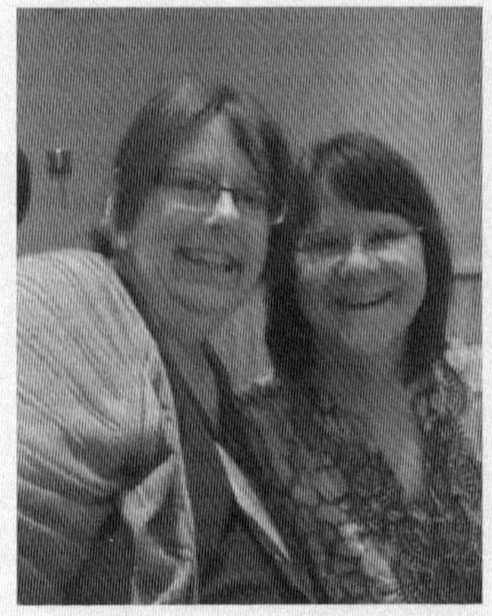

Cheri Grant (left) and Gail Tully of Spinning Babies® (right).

PREFACE

YOU MAY HAVE THE most powerful tool in your hands for childbirth! But having a peanut ball is not the same as knowing how to use one. It's possible to provide little usefulness, or worse—do harm by not knowing how to use the peanut ball correctly.

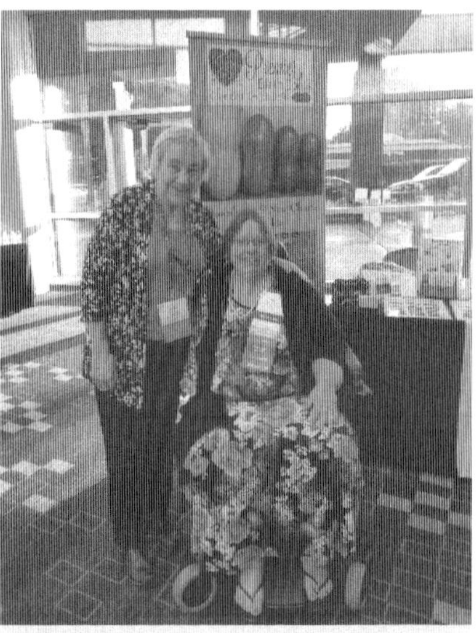

Penny Simkin and Cheri Grant
Thank you, Penny, for your inspiration.

I was first introduced to peanut balls in the 1980s as a Labor and Delivery nurse. At that time, we only used them in the Straddle Position, but I knew they were a great tool in helping progress labor.

Peanut balls have now become a widely accepted birth tool, and it's my mission to help educate more people about their effectiveness and evidence-based improvements to Labor and Delivery. In fact, my goal is to have peanut balls in every Labor and Delivery room!

It has been the biggest thrill to see peanut balls become a widely accepted tool, and I hope this book will help make peanut ball information accessible to even more people around the world.

Disclaimer

Please discuss with your doctor, midwife, nurse, or doula before performing any of the positions shown in this book. Do not attempt any positions that make any current health conditions worse. Seek help from a medical professional to perform positions in a safe environment, using proper body mechanics in choosing a position. While the positions covered in this book are used and recommended by the author and contributors, new positions are being invented all the time as the awareness and use of the peanut ball continues to grow around the world.

INTRODUCTION

I HAVE BEEN IN Labor and Delivery Maternity care for 50 years as a nurse, ICEA childbirth educator, and DONA doula. I started in Maternity at age 11, in a small rural hospital in Oklahoma that had only one labor room. Dr. Olson, who delivered me as a baby, said, "You do not want to work In OB. Come with me and I will show you why!" He took me to the hospital to be with a mom in labor and birth. As she breathed with each contraction, I felt more and more compassion for her. It was 1970, before dads were allowed in the delivery room. I volunteered to carry a pager and be on call 24/7. When we had a mom come in for labor, I would be paged out of school. I stayed with the mom until the baby was born, even if it took 24 hours. This is the moment I knew I wanted to work in Labor and Delivery.

In the 1980s when I was working in Labor and Delivery, I went to the physical therapy department and borrowed a peanut ball to facilitate my patient's delivery. Then 25 years later, I began using the peanut ball in various postions besides the straddle postion. Nurses and doulas in other Labor and Delivery departments began using the peanut ball with their patients in increasing frequency, because they worked. They sped up labor and my hunch was they prevented Cesarean Delivery.

Peanut balls have found homes in diverse childbirth locations and I made it an aim to teach others the remarkable improvements to the birthing experience gained through peanut ball use. I also worked to make peanut balls available to hospitals, nurses, doulas, and childbirth supporters. My passion for coming alongside laboring women to enrich and improve the birth experience was a driving force toward my contributions—or legacy—in advancing peanut ball use. In practice, informal research, publications, videos, podcasts, and presentations, I have promoted safe and effective use of peanut balls.

Over the years, I have found there is a great deal of misinformation about peanut balls. I wrote this book to widely share correct and evidence-based information about peanut balls so our industry has the necessary information for correct use during labor.

My goal is that you learn the basics of using the peanut ball in Labor and Delivery settings. I will share information about peanut ball safety, contraindications, and how to determine the correct size of peanut ball for your client.

You will learn new positions including Flying Cowgirl, Rock the Boat, and Park Bench. I will help you understand basic and advanced labor and pushing techniques that can be used with the peanut ball.

Most importantly, you will be able to differentiate internal or external rotation of the client's femur or thigh bone to use in relation to where the baby is in the pelvis inlet, midpelvis, and outlet with the peanut ball. You will learn which peanut ball positions to use to assist and facilitate the baby's descent through the stations.

To be more effective, each nurse should attend a hands-on in-service training and skills lab competency checklist. *A study done on peanut balls showed there was a 6 percent decrease in the cesarean rate after nurses were trained on peanut ball (Palladino 2019,* S28-S29). It is so important to share the correct information, and Premier Birth Tools and Authorized Peanut Ball Trainers makes that easy!

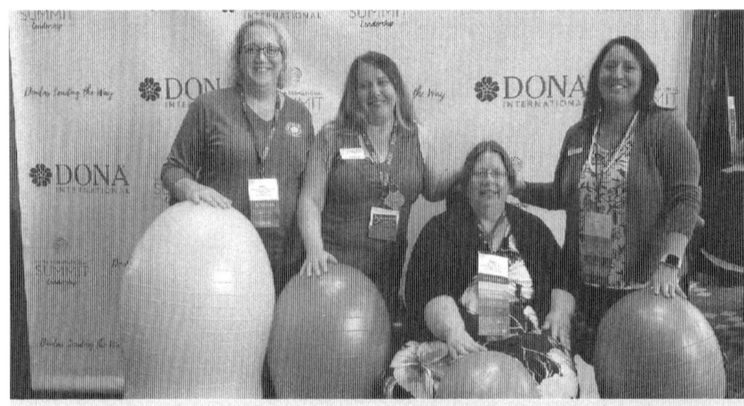

Authorized Peanut Ball Trainers:
Amy Emerson, Heather Turner, Cheri Grant, and Melissa Harley

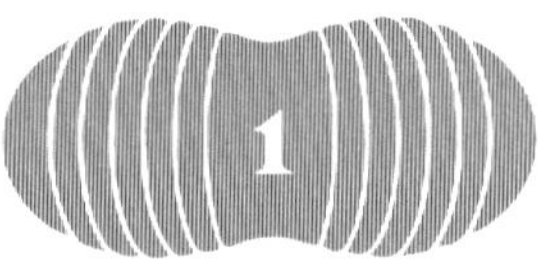

HISTORY OF PEANUT BALLS

"This peanut ball tool should be available for every delivery. It should be taught to every labor nurse, the same as teaching how to apply fetal monitoring devices."

—Nona Barnett, labor and delivery nurse and Authorized Peanut Ball Trainer, Oregon

I WAS FIRST INTRODUCED to peanut balls in the 1980s as a Labor and Delivery nurse when they were first used during birth. A client was in labor but could not get comfortable. I brought in the peanut ball and I had her staddle it (similar to picture on the following page). The client's husband sat behind her. As she leaned into his chest, she immediately relaxed. Feeling secure and supported, she stopped fighting the contractions and let her body work. The love hormone—oxytocin—kicked in, the baby moved in a better position, and she gave birth to a beautiful baby. At that time, we only used the peanut ball in the Straddle Position, but I knew they were a great tool in helping to progress labor.

The use of the peanut ball in Labor and Delivery can be traced back to the round birth ball, which was created in the early 1960s by Aquilino Cosan in Italy. The round birth ball was first introduced in the United States in Labor and Delivery units in the 1980s by Polly Perez, RN, and Penny Simkin, PT. Sitting on the round birth ball became popular in maintaining an upright position, which assisted in the gravitational descent of the fetal head through the pelvis (Perez 2000, 1–2). It also allowed gentle motion, which tipped and changed the pelvis in ways that facilitated fetal descent.

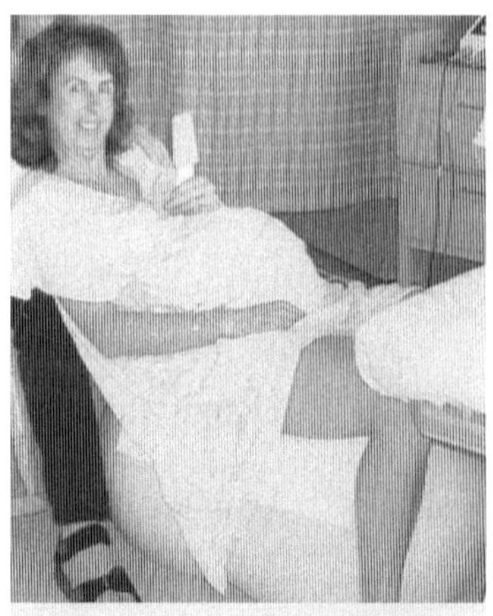

Photo courtesy of Polly Perez RN

In the 1990s, doulas and nurses were taught how to use the peanut ball by Polly Perez, RN. At that time, clients only used the Straddle Position as they found its inward sloping oblong shape cradled the abdomen and provided increased control and stability, while its ringed grooves provided increased traction. During this time, round birth balls were widely used. It would take years to recognize peanut balls were extremely beneficial during Labor and Delivery in different positions. In one study "64% of women using the peanut ball stated it helped facilitate progress of labor. 71% would recommend use of the peanut ball" (Payton, 2015).

In 2010, I started to use the peanut ball in different positions. I was with a client who had an epidural and was in the Side-Lying Position. The client's labor progressed slowly, because of the position of the baby's head. I knew if I propped the client's top leg on several pillows, it would help the baby turn to the correct position. Unfortanately, the plastic hospital pillows kept slipping from between her legs. I got a peanut ball, placed it between the client's legs, and it easily stayed in place. The client went from 4 cm to ready to push in 34 minutes. I still remember that day. The client was excited to meet her beautiful baby and I found a new peanut ball position—the Tuck—that worked well. Over the next several years, many more positions were created and I learned how the peanut ball helped speed up labor.

In 2011, the peanut ball gained popularity and wider use in Labor and Delivery in different positions. I remember the first time I brought it to a small-town hospital, in Owasso, Oklahoma, and taught a few nurses how to use it. They could not believe the results. (See the unpublished research chapter.) The peanut ball use has become my passion. *Childbirth Graphics* in 2014 named me the "Peanut Ball Lady." I believe peanut balls should be in every Labor and Delivery, birthing center, and midwives' hands to use during labor to assist in faster labors and help babies to get in better position for labor. The improvements promote mother and baby well-being.

In 2022, the peanut ball is a widely accepted birth tool used in Labor and Delivery in several positions, which will be demonstrated in more detail throughout this book.

THE TIMELINE OF PEANUT BALLS

- **1980s** — Europe and United States began using peanut balls in the Straddle Position in limited areas
- **1990s** — Doulas, childbirth educators, Labor and Delivery nurses were trained in the Straddle Position
- **2010** — I personally started to use the peanut ball in other positions with clients
- **2011** — Use with epidurals; Tussy and Botsio's first study; first citation in the Side-Lying Position
- **2014** — I introduced seven new peanut ball positions at the LAMAZE/DONA Conference
- **2014** — I published the seven original peanut ball positions in *International Doula Magazine*
- **2014** — At this time, there were only 3 citations of peanut ball articles worldwide
- **2015** — Authorized Peanut Ball Trainers began teaching peanut ball workshops
- **2015** — Official Peanut Ball Ambassadors began assisting the goal of getting peanut balls in more hospitals
- **2017** — Peanut balls started to be used around the world in 15 countries
- **2019** — I presented 40 new peanut ball techniques at the GOLD Perinatal International Conference and the DONA International Conference
- **2020** — Peanut balls gained exposure with over 42 citations of peanut ball articles and posters
- **2022** – As of publishing this book, new positions continue to be created. This book contains more than 50 positions

GUIDELINES ON PEANUT BALLS USE AND CARE

There are several items to consider when using peanut balls. Each of these guidelines will be discussed more in-depth throughout the book.

Guiding Principles About Peanut Balls

- Peanut balls are available in several sizes and it's important to have the right size for the client and position. Only 70 cm peanut balls are used to sit while straddling the ball. One size does not fit all clients.
- Always store peanut balls off the ground and keep away from sharp objects.
- Peanut ball height should be checked every three months to ensure proper inflation.
- Peanut balls should be protected during labor and birth with a covering.
- Peanut balls should be cleaned after each use.
- Peanut balls do have some contraindications when used in labor and birth. Check that client does not have one of these contraindications before use.
- I will present more than 50 peanut ball positions including basic and advanced positions.
- It's important to pay attention to baby's position when using the peanut ball. There are peanut ball positions for when baby is above the inlet, in the midplevis, or in the outlet.
- Peanut balls can be used during pushing to facilitate second stage.
- Peanut balls can be used both with or without an epidural in a hospital, birthing center, or at a home birth.

In 2020, we just started using the peanut ball in my nursing practice. I work in a rural 25-bed critical-access hospital where we do between 6–16 deliveries a month.

Maria Dow, nurse, Montana

Peanut balls are an important, low-tech tool that are very effective in facilitating the birth of a baby. It is important to learn how to use them correctly with clients.

TYPES OF PEANUT BALLS

There are several sizes of peanut balls: 40 cm, 45 cm, 50 cm, 55 cm, 60 cm, and 70 cm. However, the most common sizes are 40 cm, 50 cm, 60 cm, and 70 cm, and most hospitals carry only 40 cm and 50 cm. All four sizes should be available at every hospital.

Most Common Sizes

- **40 cm:** For a petite client or those with shorter legs
- **50 cm:** Most common size and used for most clients
- **60 cm:** For tall clients
- **70 cm:** Used only to sit while straddling the ball

Only a 70 cm Peanut Ball can be used to straddle or sit on, and women should use bare feet or grip-soled socks for safety (Grant 2021, 4).

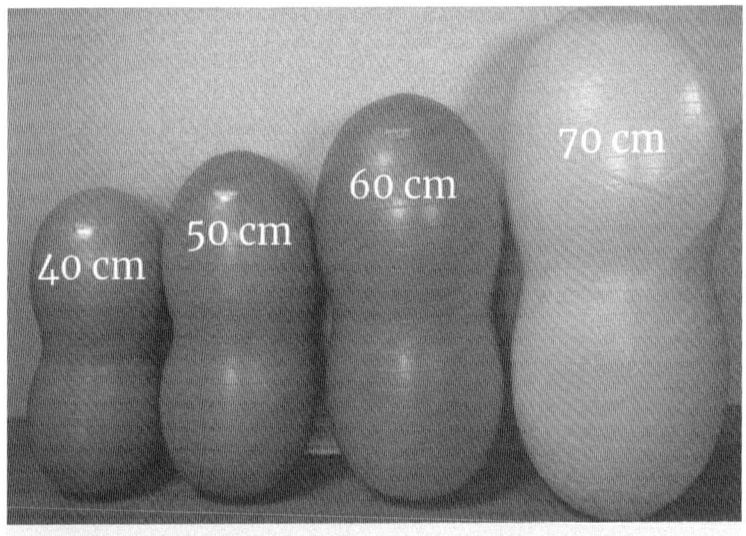

Four most common sizes. *Photo © Premier Birth Tools LLC*

Peanut Ball Composition

The peanut ball should be latex free, burst resistant, and medical grade. Check the brand you intend to purchase to make sure these requirements are all met. Medical grade peanut balls are thicker, made for multiuse, and are burst resistant. Be aware that some brands are thinner and only made for single use.

Peanut Ball Coloring

It's important to note that the coloring of peanut balls does not correlate with size, as different brands will offer different colors in different sizes. One brand may have a 50 cm blue peanut ball and another brand will sell a green 50 cm peanut ball. *Confirm the correct size of peanut ball, not the color.*

Types of Peanut Balls and Sizes

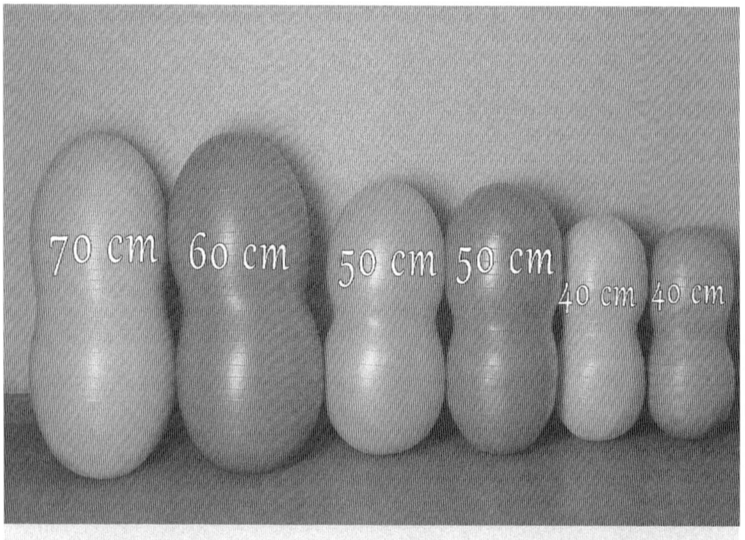

Different brands shown for comparison. *Photo © Premier Birth Tools LLC*

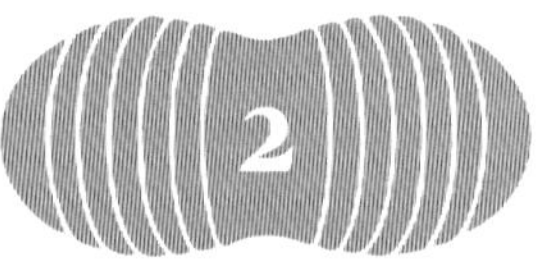

CARE OF PEANUT BALLS

"Our nursing staff has embraced the peanut balls. I purchased three for the unit and shortly afterwards ten more were bought. Nurses were fighting over the balls!"

—Wendy Wagner, OBGYN, New Jersey

PEANUT BALL STORAGE

PEANUT BALLS SHOULD BE kept away from sharp objects, direct sunlight, and high temperatures. If kept above 80 degrees, the peanut ball material will begin to deteriorate. Storage at room temperature is optimal. Always store peanut balls off the ground to prevent them from puncturing.

Tips to Properly Store Peanut Balls

- Hang with a peanut ball strap from a hook on a wall
- Hang with a peanut ball cover handle, a sheet, or rebozo tied around the ball
- Store on a shelf in a clean utility equipment room or in a closet
- Place in a cloth laundry bag and hang from IV pole
- Use a wall-storage system
- Place on a chair, in the tub, on a table, or on a cart
- *Never* place peanut balls in a warmer

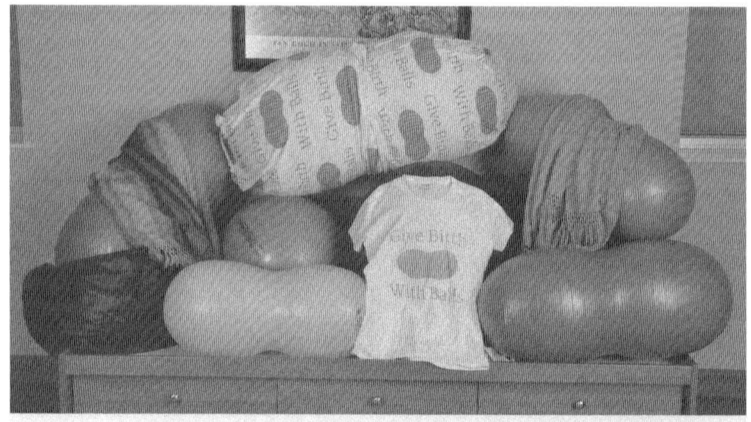

Store off the ground. *Photo © Premier Birth Tools LLC*

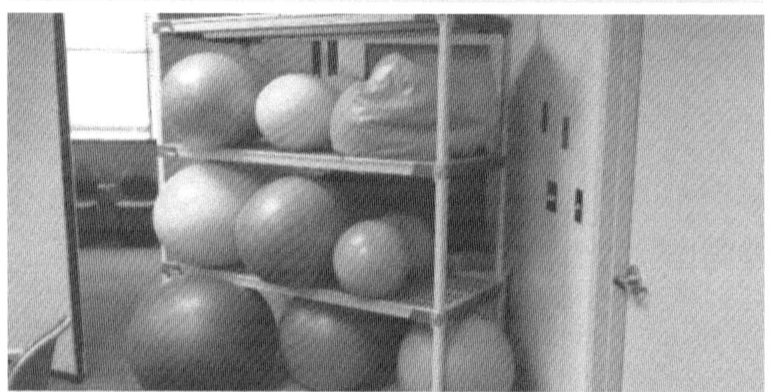

Store on a storage cart.
Photo © Premier Birth Tools LLC

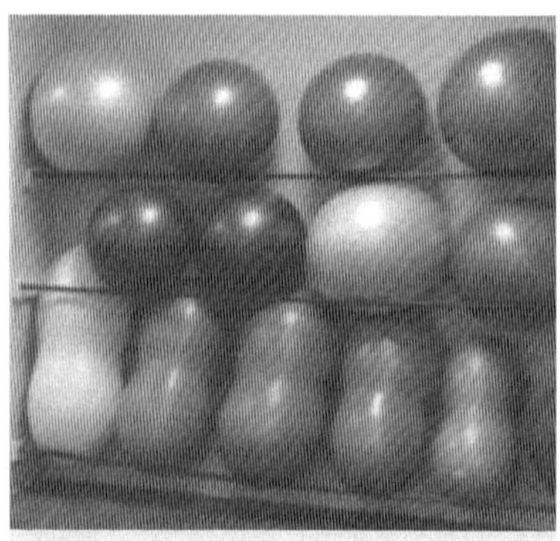

Store on a rack.
Photo courtesy of Breath Birth & Wellness

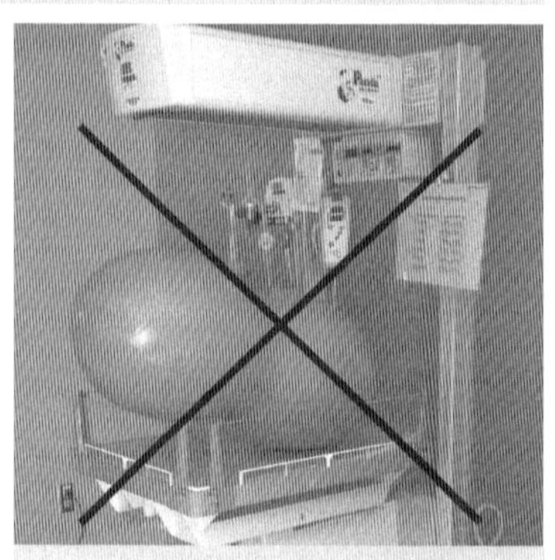

***Never* store in a warmer.**
Photo © Pre mier Birth Tools LLC

INFLATION OF PEANUT BALLS

Carefully read the peanut ball instructions and measure the peanut ball correctly when inflated. When first inflating, fill the ball at room temperature to 80 percent on the first day. On the second day, fill to the measurement on the ball and make sure not to overinflate.

Usually, the measurement is from the top of the peanut ball at the plug to the waist of the peanut ball. (See examples below.) Check peanut ball height every three months to ensure they are still properly inflated. Inflation measurements will depend on the brand, so refer to the instructions that came with your peanut ball.

To keep peanut balls properly inflated, they will need to be replaced every one to two years, depending on usage and condition.

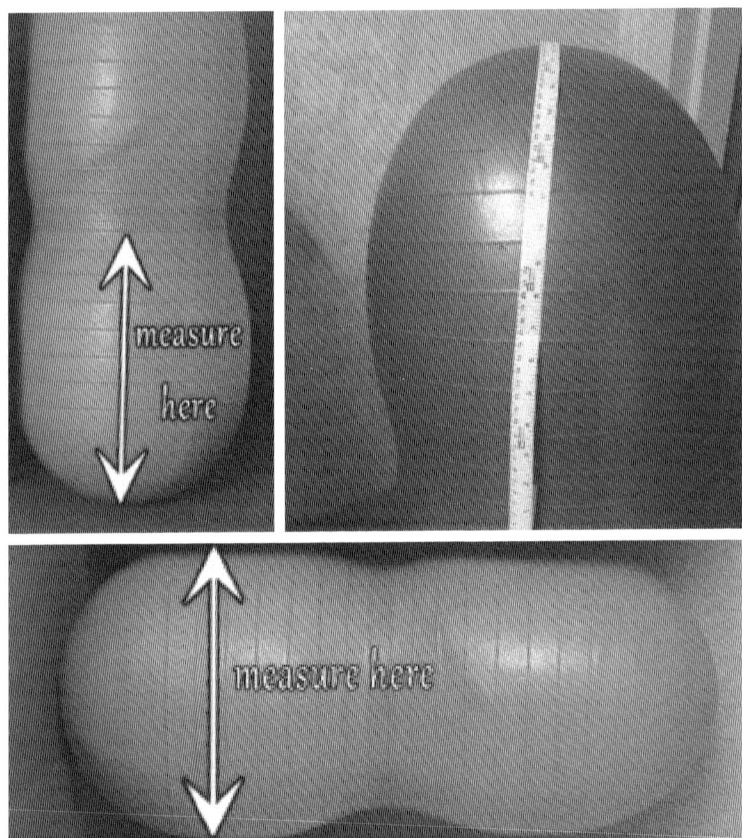

Each brand is measured differently. *Photos © Premier Birth Tools LLC*

COVERING THE PEANUT BALL

Peanut balls should be protected with a covering during use. Covering options include:

- Patient gown tied in two places with a blue pad chux underpad on top of the gown (a trash bag can also be used first then the gown)
- Flat sheet held with monitor belts and a blue pad chux underpad on top
- Flat sheet held with an abdominal binder and a blue pad chux underpad on top
- Fitted sheet
- Bath blanket
- Pillowcase pulled over each side, overlapping the middle
- Peanut ball cover
- Paper gown that wasn't used on a delivery table
- "Sterile leggings" that weren't used on a delivery table

Note: *Taping a sheet will leave a residue on the ball that will deteriorate over time. If you use tape, make sure to tape the sheet to the sheet and not the peanut ball.*

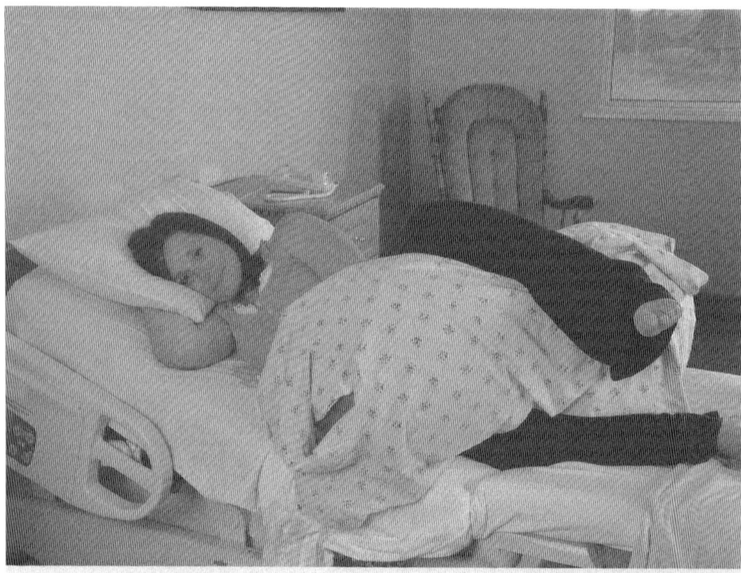

Cover peanut ball with a patient gown. *Photo © Premier Birth Tools LLC*

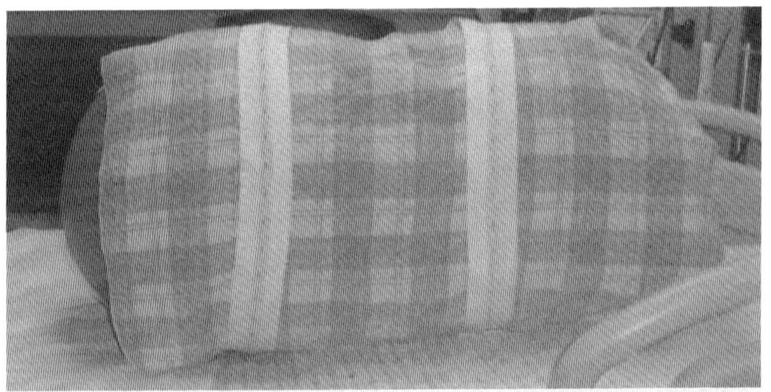

Cover peanut ball with a waterproof pad.

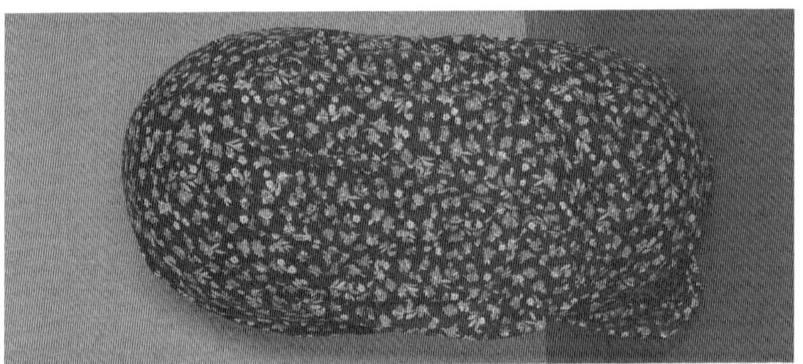

Cover peanut ball with a commercial ball cover.

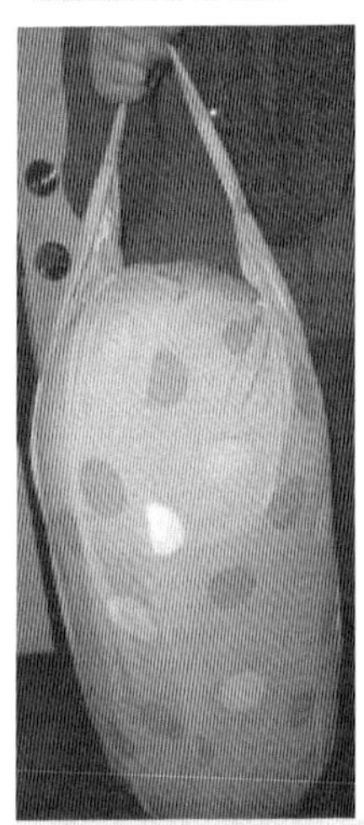

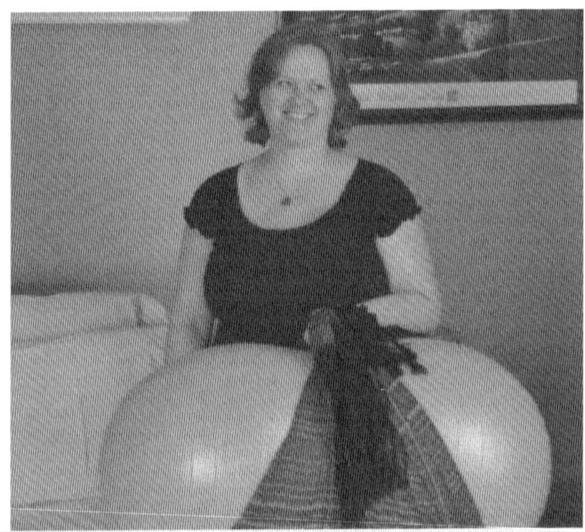

Carry your peanut ball. *Photos © Premier Birth Tools LLC*

CLEANING THE PEANUT BALL

Peanut balls should be cleaned after each use. Many types of cleaning solutions are available, but always consult your specific peanut ball's manufacturers guide for instructions. **Note:** *Peanut balls will become more discolored as they are cleaned.*

Ways to Clean a Peanut Ball

- Soap and water
- Water and vinegar
- Sani wipes or hospital grade wipes
- Rinse and scrub with disinfectant in the shower

Note: *Do not use bleach on peanut balls; it will degrade the material quickly.*

Creating a Clean/Dirty System

A clean/dirty system is necessary so nurses can quickly determine if a peanut ball has been cleaned and is ready for use. Here are some suggestions:

- Place in a clean, cloth laundry bag or a trash bag (make sure peanut balls are very dry before placing in the bag)
- Store on a shelf in a utility room, in the closet of the Labor and Delivery room, or in laundry bag hanging on an IV pole
- Designate with a sticker that says "clean" on the storage bag

Note: *Low quality peanut balls cleaned properly will not maintain their quality over time.*

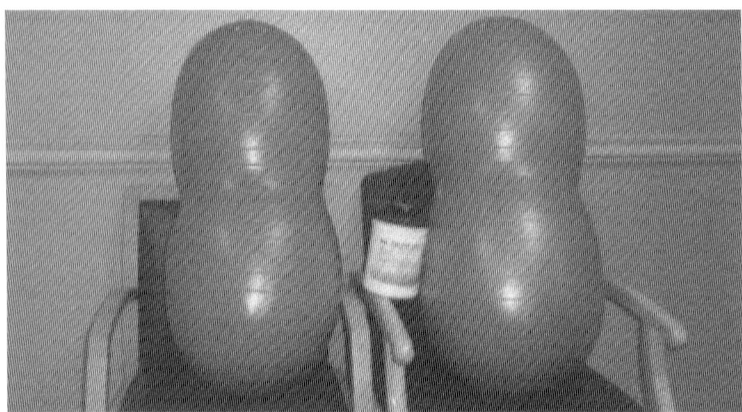

New ball (left) and cleaned ball (right). *Photo © Premier Birth Tools LLC*

TOWELS AND STIRRUPS TO SUPPORT PEANUT BALLS

When clients feel like they need to hold the peanut ball in place, they stay more tensed. A well-supported peanut ball helps the client deeply relax, which assists in labor progress. Here are some recommendations to stabilize the peanut ball:

At Home

- A firm couch pillow or rolled towel on both sides of the peanut ball for stabilzation

At Hospital

- Rolled towel or thin blanket
- Hospital pillows do not work as most are plastic and do a terrible job supporting peanut balls due to sliding
- Stirrups from the side of the bed provide adequate support

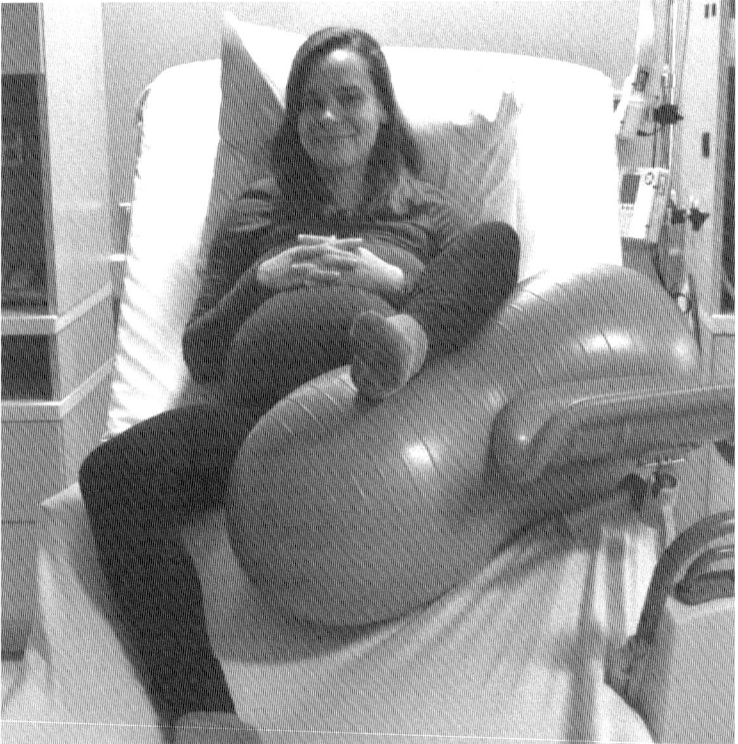

Stirrups to support the peanut ball. *Photo courtesy of Amy Bookwalter, CD*

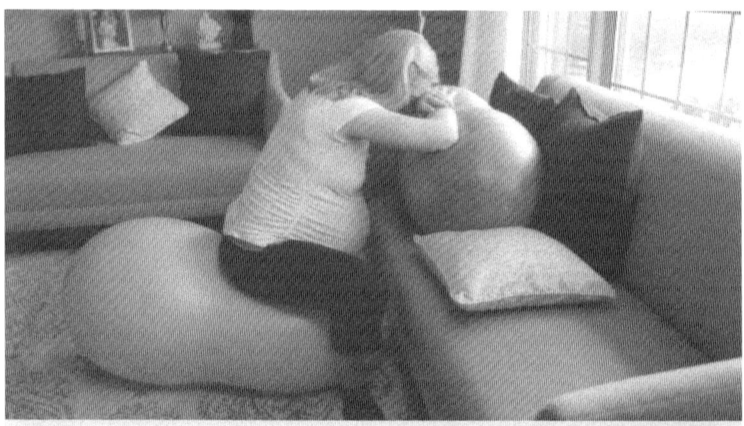

At home, use couch pillows to stabilize the peanut ball.

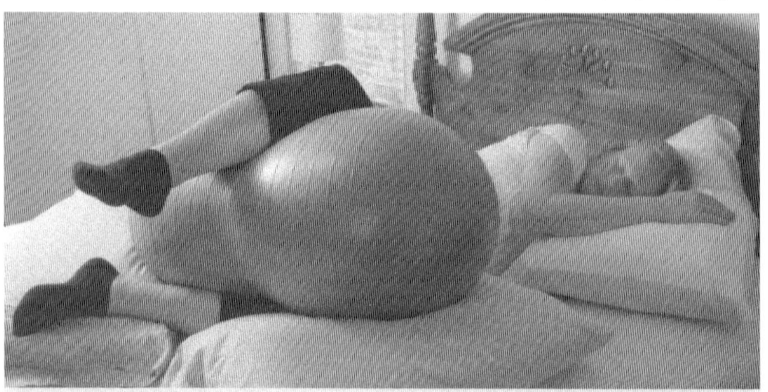

At home, pillows support peanut ball. Client can relax and not hold ball.

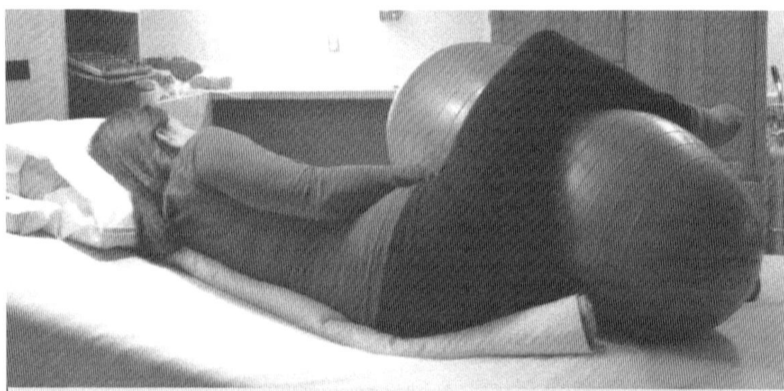

Roll towels or thin blanket in front and behind peanut ball to help stabilize.

Photos courtesy of Amy Bookwalter, CD

I attended Cheri's presentation on the peanut ball at the 2014 LAMAZE/DONA conference. After the conference, I donated a peanut ball to a couple of local hospitals. I attended a birth soon after. This client was hoping for a VBAC with her second child with a very gentle induction. Her first baby never dropped past -3 station. I explained to the doctor what I'd learned at the conference—that the peanut ball helps to shorten labors and reduces pushing time. This very young, new, and re-search savvy doctor rolled her eyes at me and said, "Well, I'd like to see those studies and I'll believe it when I see it". So, I handed her copies of the studies. This mom went from 4 cm at 11:30 am to complete at 2:50 pm and holding her baby at 3:11 pm. Her induction was using the foley overnight and resting with a peanut ball for a couple of hours in the middle of the day. The doctor became a big believer, she and the nurses love the peanut balls and the hospital has the lowest Cesarean Delivery rate in the area. It made my day and I couldn't wait to share my story. I knew Cheri would be so proud!

Amy Bookwalter, doula and Authorized
Peanut Ball Trainer, Virginia

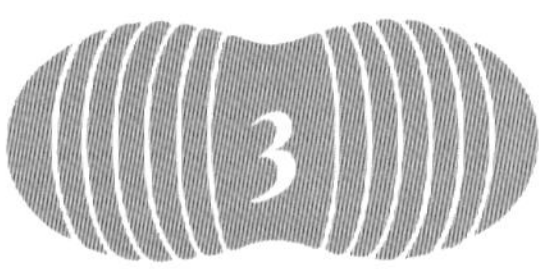

CONTRAINDICATIONS AND BEST PRACTICES FOR PEANUT BALL USE

"I found peanut balls about five years ago. I bought one for my local hospital and convinced all the nurses we need to use them. After some skepticism, they were all believers."

—Shannon Kent, doula, Connecticut

PEANUT BALLS DO HAVE some contraindications when used in labor and birth. I have listed several here, but this is not an all-inclusive list and you may find more during use. Always ask the client if they have any contraindications before offering the peanut ball to them.

CONTRAINDICATIONS FOR USE OF THE PEANUT BALL

- Previous hip or pelvis injury
- Broken hip or pelvis
- Broken symphysis or symphysis pubis dysfunction
- Active diagnosed DVT (Deep Vein Thrombosis)

Caution: *Not every peanut ball position is a good position. Let each client guide what feels right and helpful. This includes the size of peanut ball.*

Maternal comfort is most important when sizing and positioning the peanut ball. While some positions may seem awkward, they should be comfortable and facilitate fetal descent. Client limbs should always be supported; towels can help stabilize the peanut ball position.

BEST PRACTICES FOR PEANUT BALL USE

- Always support the leg and ankle without twisting or dropping
- Maintain proper body mechanics when used with an epidural and client is numb
- If clients states that the position does not feel good, listen to the client
- Change positions frequently and do not leave client in same position for more than 45 minutes to an hour (**Note:** *No problems have been reported due to this, caution in positioning is necessary*)
- Use a towel to stabilize the peanut ball
- Use the correct size of peanut ball for the client in a selected position. If the ball is too large it places too much abduction of hip joint and causes guarding, not relaxing

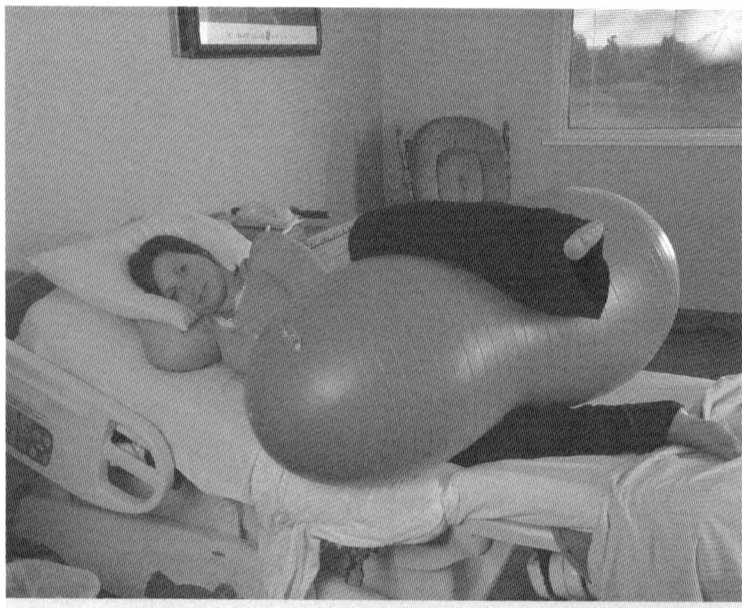

This size is too big for this client. *Photo © Premier Birth Tools LLC*

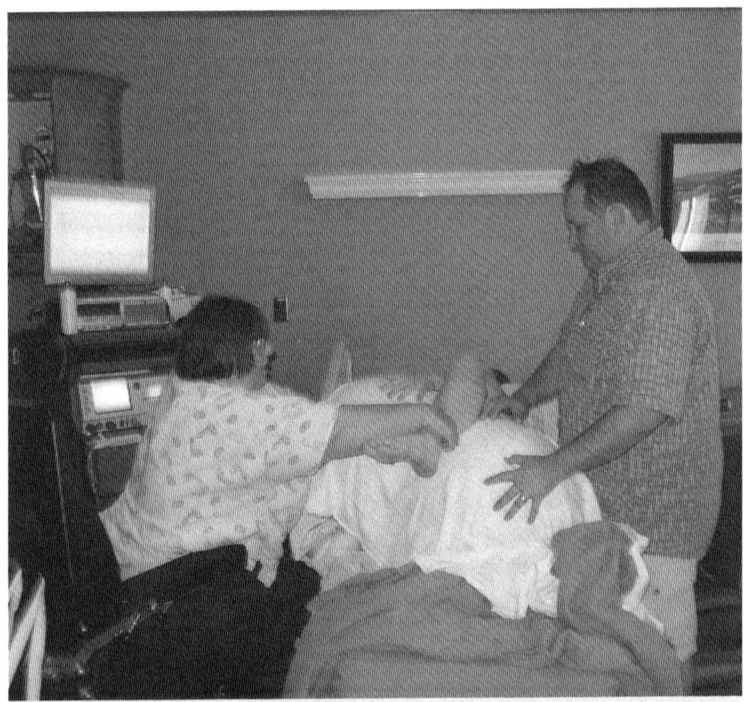

Support the client's leg without twisting.
Cheri with client, using a peanut ball. *Photo © Premier Birth Tools LLC*

> *I have loved implementing peanut balls into practice and seeing the success. Doctors, who are at first skeptical, see the change and then become believers.*
>
> Amy Swales, nurse, Mississippi

COMFORT AND RELAXATION WITH PEANUT BALLS

It is important that clients feel confortable when using a peanut ball position during labor or pushing. Nikki Zerfas, nurse and Spinning Babies® Approved Trainer from Washington, says it the best:

> *I think we sometimes get so focused on being in the "right" position—even though it may be awkward or new—that the birthing person is left tense and actively holding the ball and the position. I like to point out that the birthing person should not need to focus their energy or muscle on holding the ball in place. I find that part of positioning with a ball is to support the ball (and the person) with pillows, folded blankets, or a helper so the birthing person is comfortable and can relax into the position.*

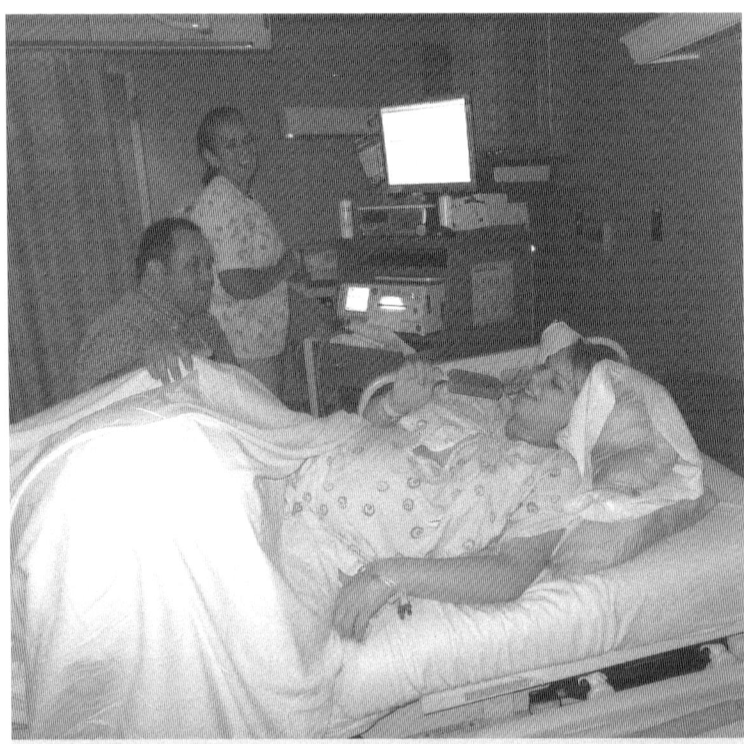

Comfort and relaxation with a peanut ball. *Photo © Premier Birth Tools LLC*

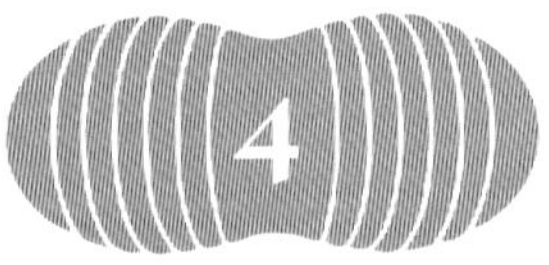

CORRECT SIZE OF PEANUT BALLS

"In November of 2016 I had a call from a hospital in Tennessee. The Labor and Delivery unit had moved to a new floor, but their peanut balls were nowhere to be found. All the nurses, doctors, and midwives were upset because they knew how much of a difference peanut balls made for women in labor. The nurse manager called and asked if we could supply one overnight. Of course, we said yes! We were thrilled about how much they loved their peanut balls!"

—Cheri Grant, RN

CORRECT SIZE OF PEANUT BALLS

AFTER SIZING HUNDREDS OF clients, I have found that one size does *not* fit all. Peanut balls should be fitted based on your client's height, but also on the position being used. If the peanut ball is too large, it places too much torque in lateral aspect during abduction of hip joint, causing guarding and not relaxing. If the peanut ball is too small, it is not as effective.

Here are our guidelines based on height:

- 40 cm for a petite client or those with shorter legs
- 50 cm ball for average clients
- 60 cm for tall clients
- 70 cm is only recommended for sitting and not to be used in the Side-Lying Position.

A client might also use all four peanut ball sizes during labor depending on the position. For example, one client may use a 40 cm ball in Semi-Sitting, 50 cm ball with Tuck, and a 60 cm ball for Forward Leaning.

Note: *It's also important to try to fit a peanut ball, before an epidural, in order to feel which size is comfortable in different positions.*

Learn More

Authorized Peanut Ball Trainer Heather Turner created a video to demonstrate the correct sizing of a peanut ball. You can find it on the YouTube channel Your Birth - DONA Certified Birth Doula and Lamaze Childbirth Educator, titled "Sizing the Peanut Ball Part 1."

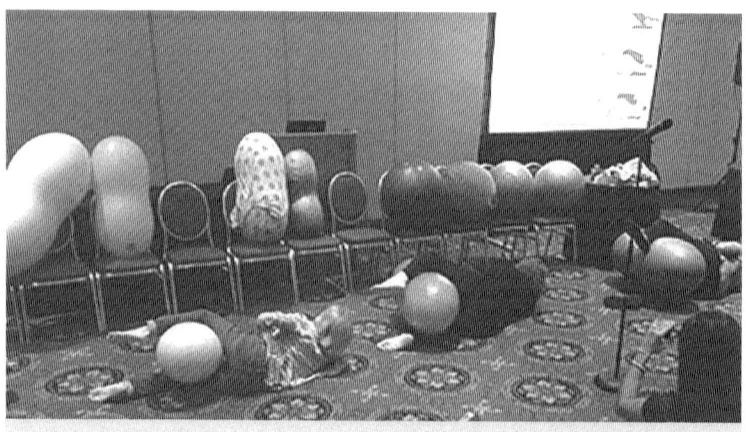

Different size peanut ball for each client. *Photo © Premier Birth Tools LLC*

A client was being induced and when I arrived, she was 1 cm after over 12 hours of Pitocin. Nurse was using Side-Lying with a peanut ball, but using it incorrectly. I adjusted [the client's] position and she began to soften and thin. Dilation happened all at once hours later, but the immediate results of correctly using the peanut ball were amazing.

Kristen Mason, doula, Maryland

Checking for Correct Fit

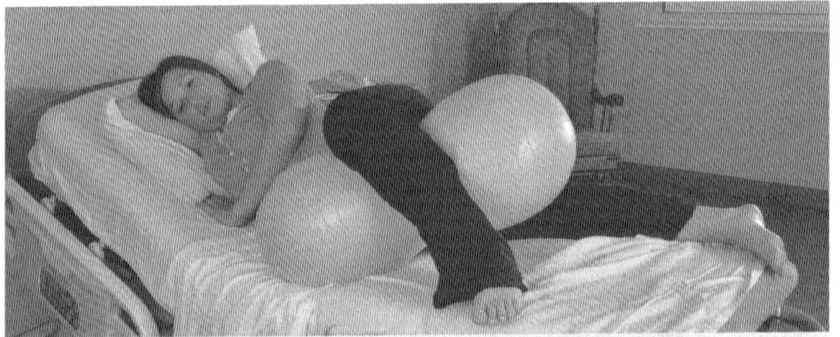

Incorrect fit for this client. Ankle hangs over ball, close outlet.

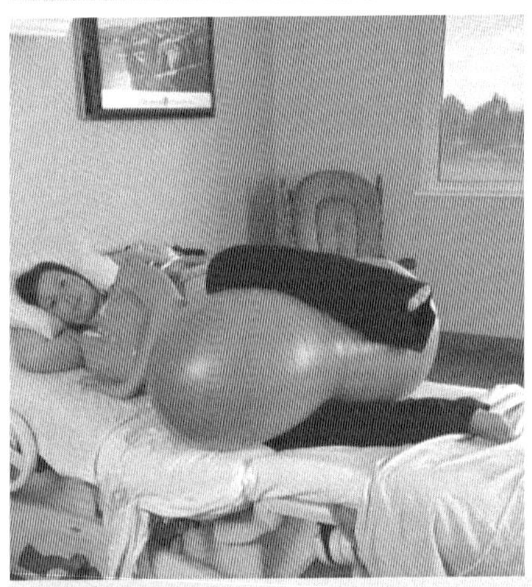

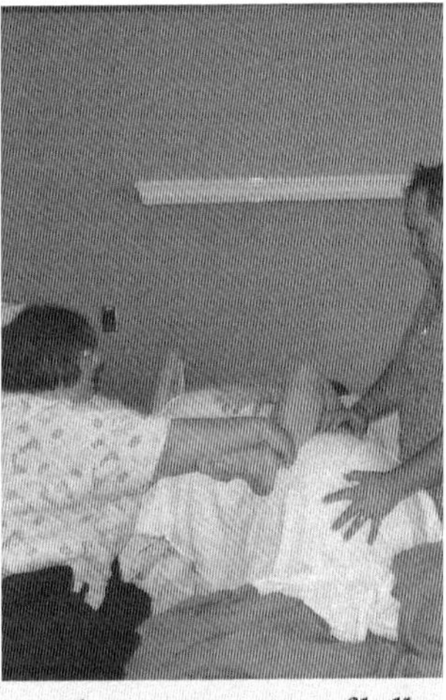

Correct fit for this client. Ankle is not hanging, rather resting on top of ball.

Photos © Premier Birth Tools LLC

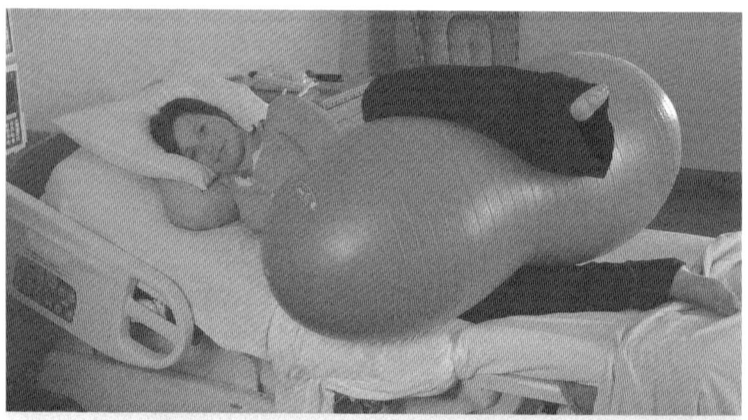

Ball is too large for this client.

Same client, different positions and different sizes of peanut balls:

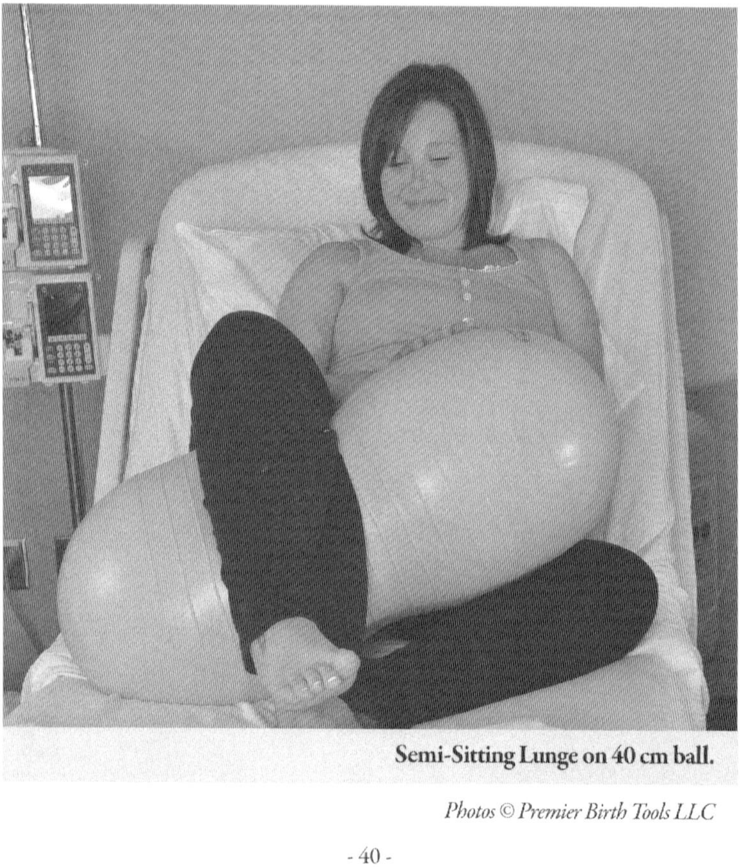

Semi-Sitting Lunge on 40 cm ball.

Photos © Premier Birth Tools LLC

We are so excited that Robin donated peanut balls to our Labor and Delivery unit. They are a tremendous help to our nurses, especially having the right size of peanut balls for their patients to use.

Amber Slaughter, nurse manager, Texas Health

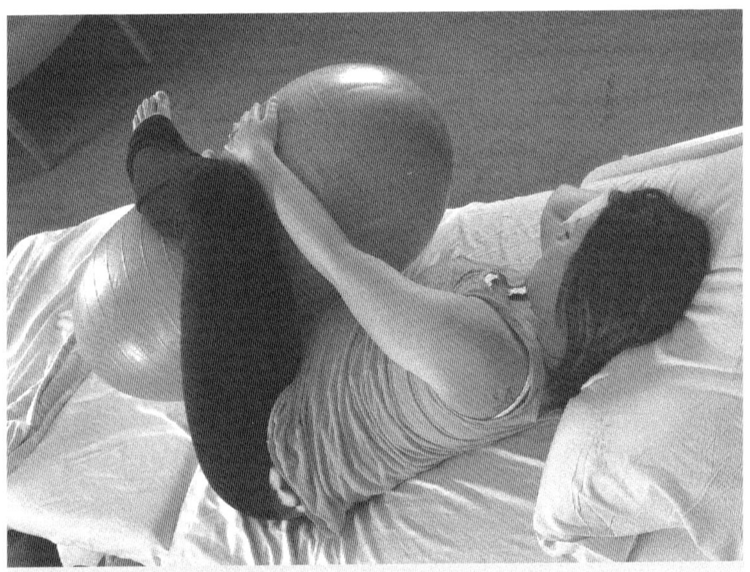

Tuck with 50 cm ball. *Photo © Premier Birth Tools LLC*

I work with a nurse who is a Peanut Ball Ambassador. We came on to our shift and I was taking care of a patient who was a multip, but was dilated to a 5 and had not made any cervical change in the last few hours. One of the nurses helped me position my patient in the Tuck Position. After an hour and a half, my patient was complete!

Olivia Haug, nurse, Missouri

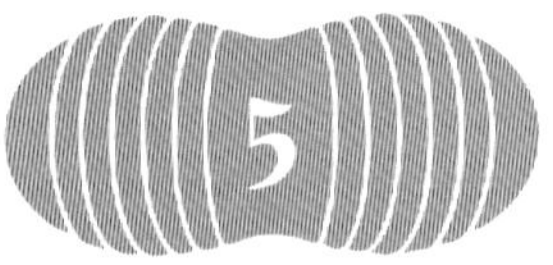

BASIC PEANUT BALL POSITIONS

"As a Labor and Delivery Nurse my favorite thing to do is celebrate births! The peanut ball is the best nurse-led tool I can use to bring to the birthday party to give to my patients the best chance of a vaginal birth. I use them every time, with every patient, and I encourage you to use them, too!"

—Hannah Ferguson, nurse, Virginia

IN A 2019 STUDY, women with an epidural, using a peanut ball were, 50 percent less likely to have a Cesarean birth. It's a powerful tool but knowing what peanut ball position to use is essential for success (Hickey 2019, 245–252).

When I first started educating nurses, midwives, and doulas on peanut ball positions in 2011, there were only seven peanut ball positions:

- Side Lying
- Tuck
- Semi-Sitting Lunge
- Forward Leaning
- Straddling
- Hands and Knees Fire Hydrant
- Pushing

Now in 2022, there are more than 50 different peanut ball positions. Many of the current peanut ball positions will be illustrated in the following chapters, but know that videos can be even more helpful. Please make sure to watch videos produced by our Authorized Peanut Ball Trainers to ensure accurate information on positions and peanut ball placement. You can visit premierbirthtools.com for more information.

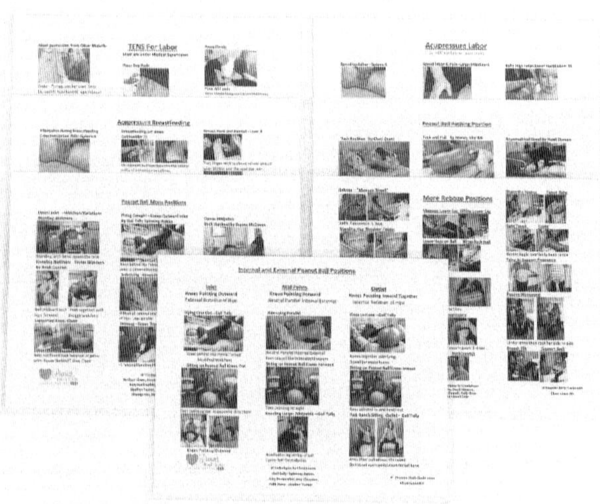

Set of 5 Peanut Ball Charts. *Photo © Premier Birth Tools LLC*

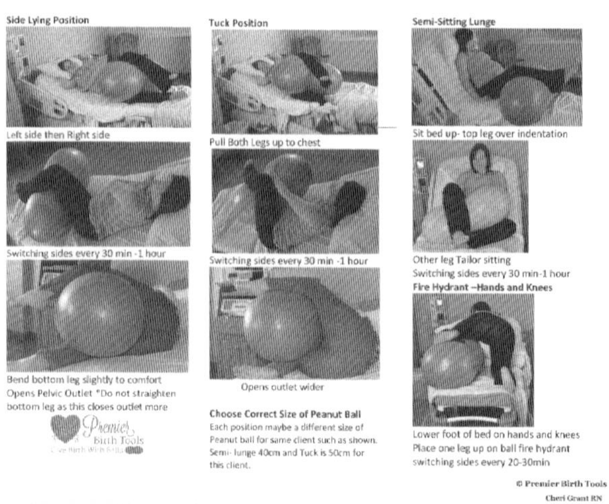

Original Peanut Ball Positions Chart. *Photo © Premier Birth Tools LLC*

Love using their position sheets for a visual aid when describing positions to clients!

Ailish McMahon-Lewis, childbirth educator and doula, Connecticut

Side-Lying Position

The Side-Lying Position, or Semi-Prone Position, is very common, especially after an epidural. The peanut ball is placed between the client's legs while lying on their side, which opens the pelvic midpelvis. Many nurses place a blanket or towel on the back of the peanut ball so it will stay in place. The clients comfort level will determine the correct placement if no epidural is present.

- Place peanut ball between client's legs, while lying on side, with the top leg over the indention
- Make sure client is turned all the way on their side. Their back should not be flat on the bed
- Turn client on each side for 30 minutes to help the baby work through the middle of the pelvis and get past the ischial spines

Note: *See Chapter 8 for detailed information.*

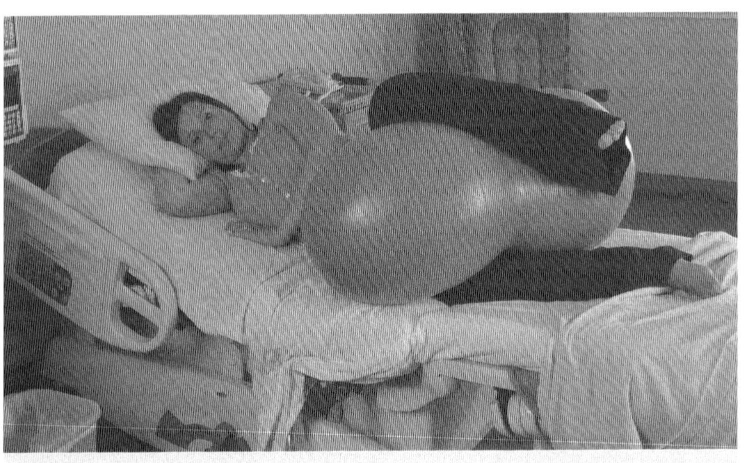

Side-Lying Position. *Photo © Premier Birth Tools LLC*

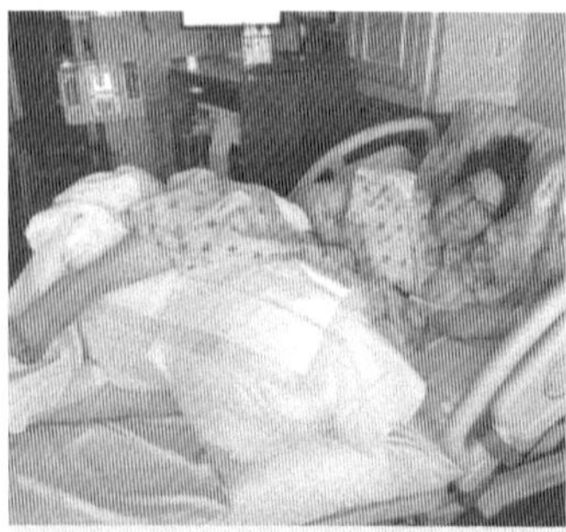

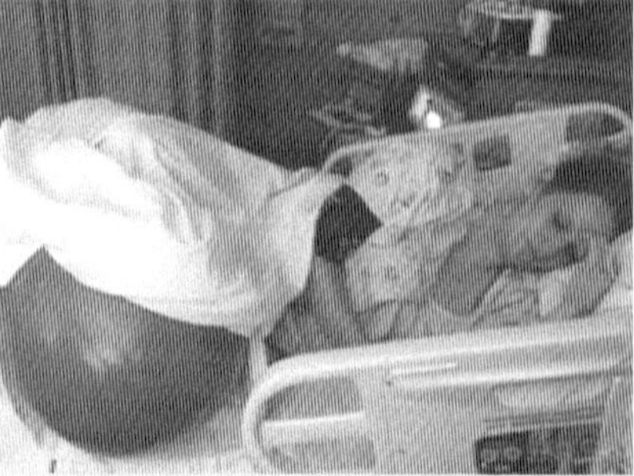

Side-Lying Position. Use a cover on peanut ball. *Photos courtesy of Sarah Coffin*

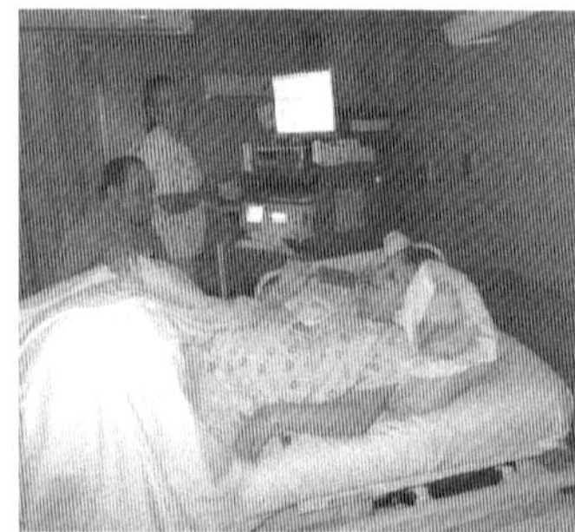

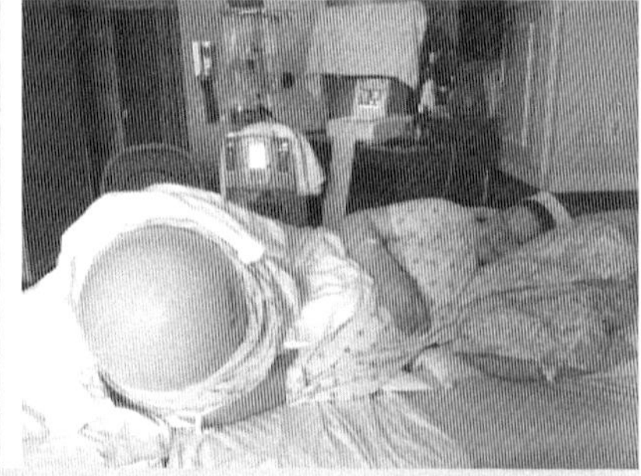

Side-Lying Position. Do not lay with back flat on bed. Turn fully on side.
Photos courtesy of Premier Birth Tools LLC (L) & Amy Emerson, RN, Doula for Birth (R).

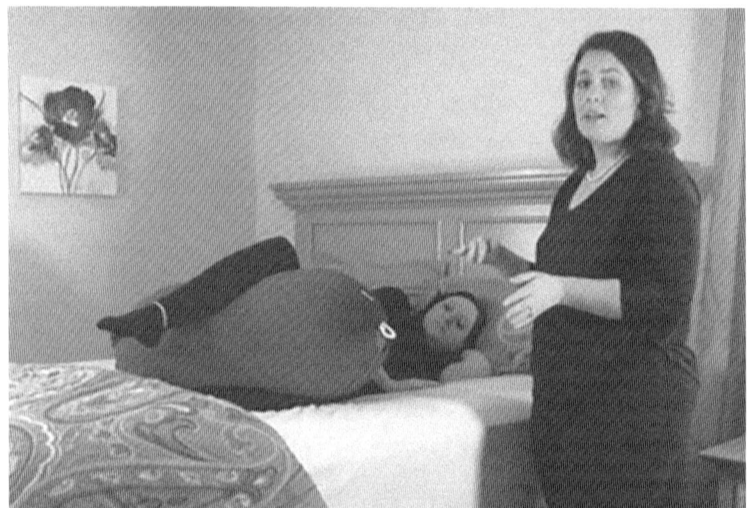

At home, Side-Lying Position.
Photos courtesy of Emma Whitlock, doula, Womb with Doula Service.

Tuck Position

By Cheri Grant, RN

The Tuck Position is one of the most important positions and allows the most efficient opening of the midpelvis. This position can assist to rotate a posterior positioned baby to a more optimal fetal position and allows the baby to descend when in the midpelvis. Tuck is also a wonderful pushing/second stage position discussed later in the book.

1. Place the peanut ball as high as possible between the client's legs with the top leg over the indention.
    - The leg under the ball should be as close to the client's chest as possible
2. Bring the peanut ball in close to the client as she is hugging it (see pictures)
    - To assist with positioning ,the bedrail can be used to hold the ball in place and a blanket can be put behind the ball.

Note: *See Chapter 9 for detailed information.*

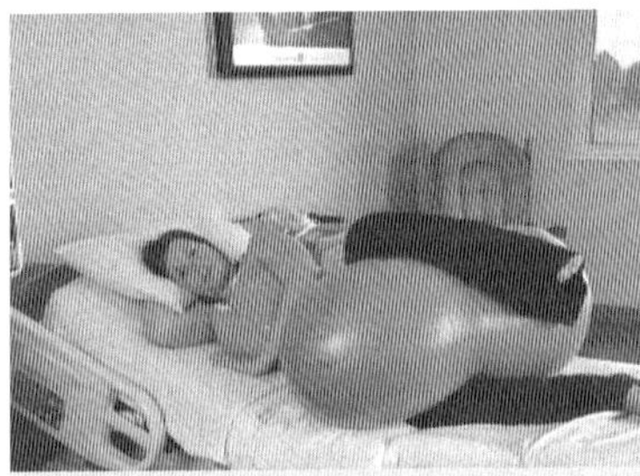

Bend lower leg close to chest.

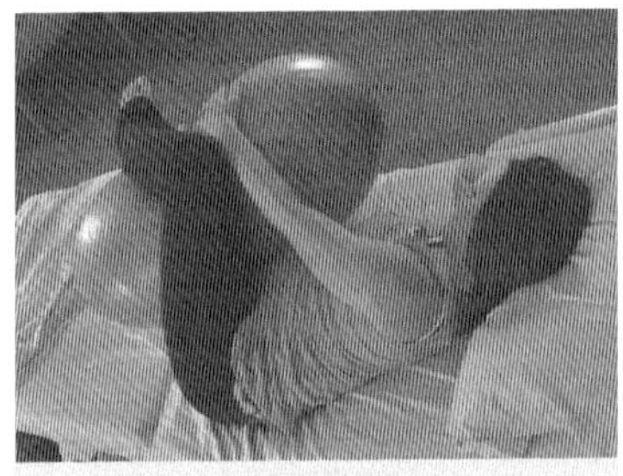

Bring ball close to chest.

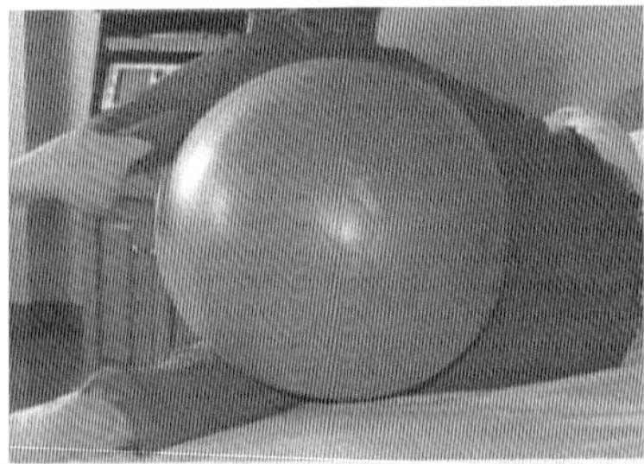

Side-Lying Positition, open.

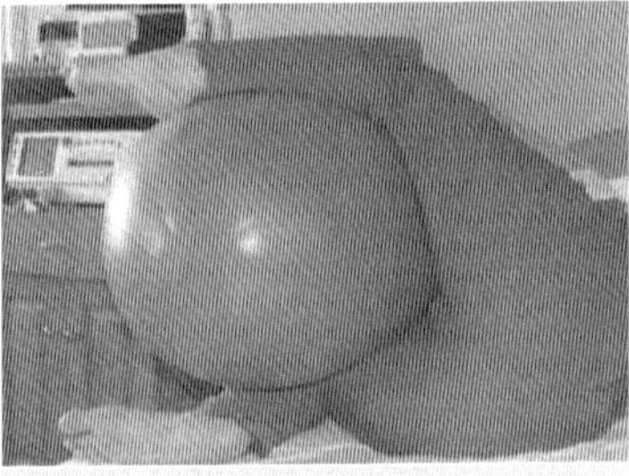

Tuck, opens even wider.

Fun Fact

How the "Tuck" Position Got Its Name

By Cheri Grant, RN

I was working with a client who was laboring with the peanut ball in the Side-Lying Position. She was making slow progress and needed more room in the pelvis. Squatting was not an option, because of an epidural, so I had her pull both knees up to the chest and hug the peanut ball. Thirty minutes later, she felt the urge to push.

"Wow, tucking that peanut ball to my chest really worked!" she said.

That is how the "Tuck" position got its name.

I'm so glad I had my 50 cm peanut ball with me while supporting a home-birthing client this week. She used the Side-Lying Position while resting, and started pushing with the Tuck Position. A beautiful baby came into the world, in a warm pool of water, [and] surrounded by loved ones.

Heather Turner, doula and Authorized Peanut Ball Trainer, California

Semi-Sitting Lunge Position

In Semi-Sitting Lunge, the client is semi-reclined on the bed with one leg over the ball, at the knee, and the other leg on bed, like a butterfly. This position encourages descent and may increase the inlet and descent if knees are out. It also promotes dilation, as the head is more applied to the cervix in an upright position. Allowing the client to lunge will open more on one side of pelvis. Do not have the client sitting straight up or it may cause too much pressure on the sacrum and coccyx.

- Head of bed up. Client is semi-reclined in bed
- One leg over the ball, at the knee, and the other leg on bed, like a butterfly

Note: *See Chapter 8 for detailed information.*

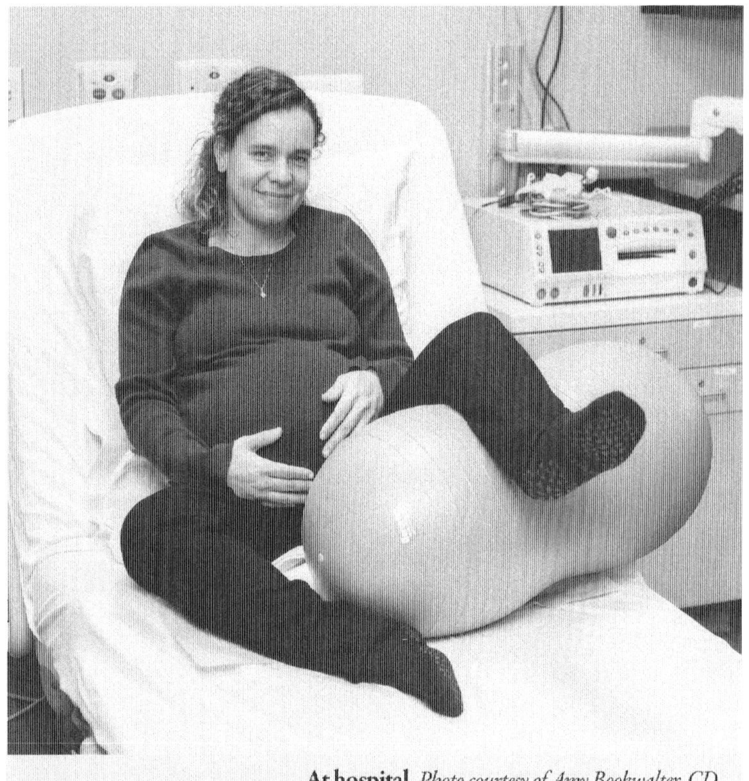

At hospital. *Photo courtesy of Amy Bookwalter, CD*

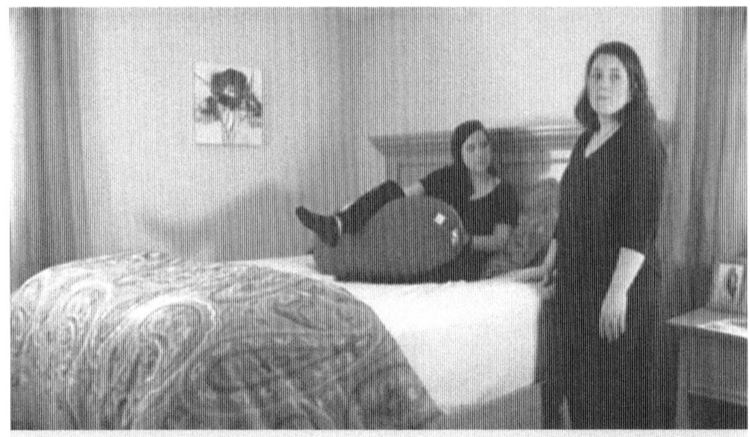

At home. *Photo courtesy of Emma Whitlock, Doula Womb Within Doula Service*

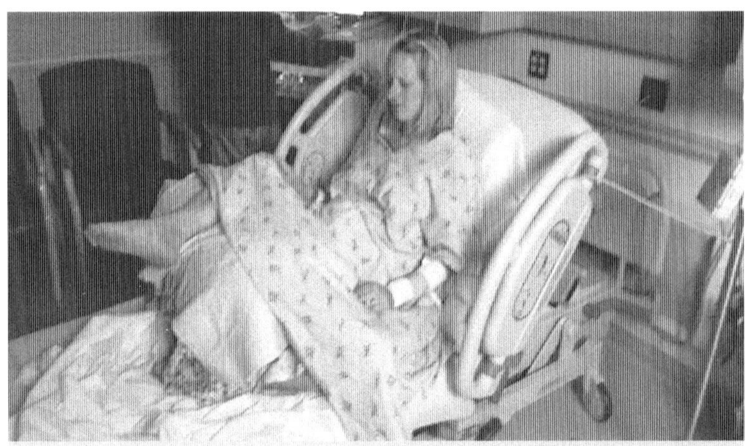

Bethany in labor. *Photo © Premier Birth Tools LLC*

When I went into labor, my midwife and nurse both recommended that I use the peanut ball in the Sitting Lunge Position. Within an hour, I went from a 4 cm to 8 cm and 15 minutes later he was born!

Kasy Wixon, doula, Oklahoma

Fire Hydrant Position

By Cheri Grant, RN

1. Place the client on hands and knees, and lower the bottom of the bed. A bean bag can be used to support the client for comfort. Scoop out hole in the bean bag, so the client is hanging the baby and it can turn to the optimal position, especially if occiput posterior. This opens half of the pelvis mid and outlet.

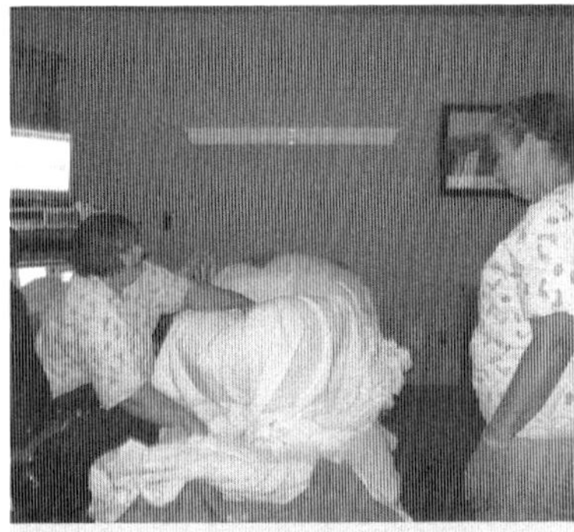

Bean bag used to support client.

2. Then place the peanut ball on the lower portion of the bed, and place the client's leg on the peanut ball in a Fire Hydrant Position or Kneeling Lunge. This position may aide in reducing an anterior cervical lip. This position also widens the midpelvis to make room for baby to rotate. For instance, if it is in an occiput transverse position. The Fire Hydrant Position is challenging for the client to keep stable. Be sure to use bed railings, people positioned beside the client, towels, or bean bag chairs to support this position.
3. Place the client on hands and knees and lower the bottom of the bed.

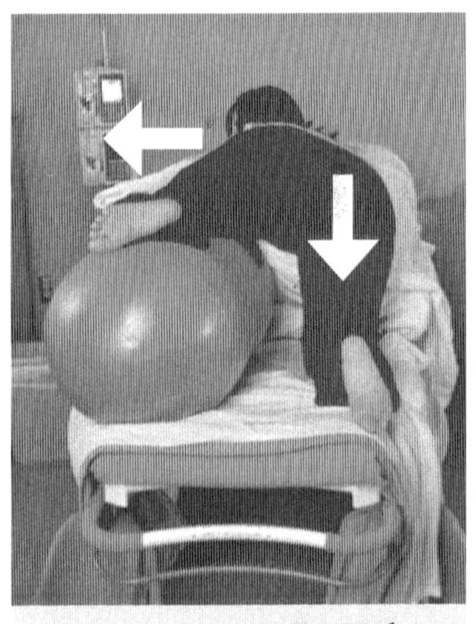

Fire Hydrant.

Photos © Premier Birth Tools LLC

Note: *See Chapter 9 for detailed information.*

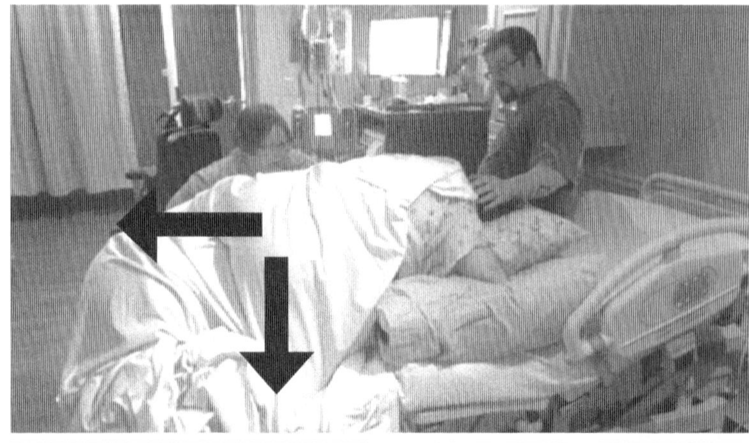

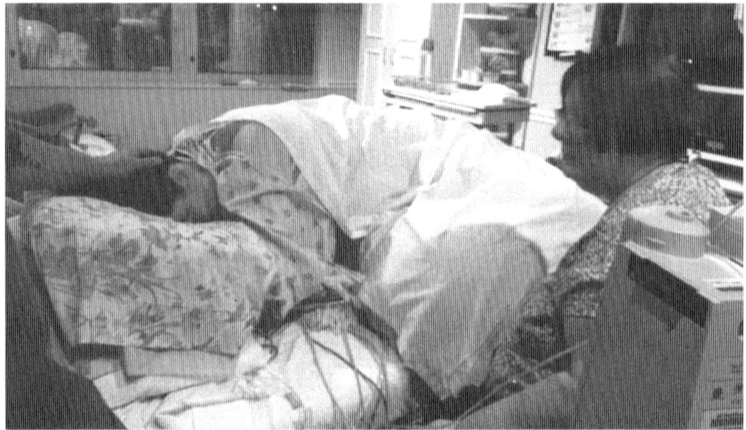

Cheri encourages client with an epidural. *Photos courtesy of Sarah Coffin*

Fun Fact

How the Position Got Its Name

By Cheri Grant, RN

I was working with a client trying to open half of the midpelivs. I knew this position could be helpful, but I was having trouble describing how to get into the postion. Finally, I whispered in the clients ear, "It's like peeing on a fire hydrant." Instantly, the client understood and was able to get in the postion. This position has also been known as the Kneeing Lunge, but many nurses and doulas have used Fire Hydrant over the years to help their clients understand the position. That is how the Fire Hydrant Position got its name.

Leaning Forward Over the Peanut Ball

Lower the bottom of the bed, then have the client lean over the peanut ball on their hands and knees. Resting on the peanut ball provides comfort and also makes sure the client is hanging the baby so it can turn to the optimal position, especially if occiput posterior or asynclitic. Leaning Forward will provide some gravity advantage and aligns the fetus with the pelvis. This position will aide in opening the inlet, mid-pelvis, or outlet, depending which way the knees are pointed (this will be discussed in a future chapter.) This position may aide in reducing an anterior cervical lip.

- Place client on hands and knees and lower the bottom of the bed
- Have client lean over the peanut ball

Note: *See Chapter 9 for detailed information*

> *My client used the peanut ball for pushing in Hands and Knees Positon. She delivered a 9 pound 14 ounce baby in less than one hour. I teach comfort measures classes at a hospital in the physical therapy department. I use their peanut ball to instruct couples how to use it in labor, with and without epidurals in place.*
>
> Sandra Hess, nurse and childbirth educator, Virginia

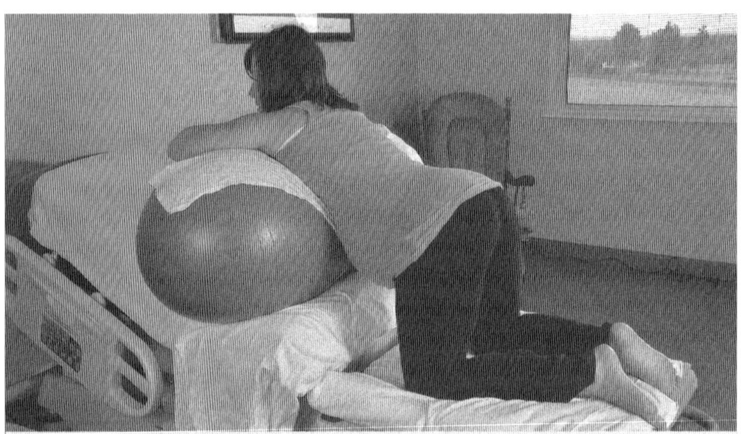

Forward-Leaning Position. *Photo © Premier Birth Tools LLC*

Sitting on the Peanut Ball Position

This position allows the client to rest, straddling the peanut ball. It also allows movement in two planes—a forward to backward movement (primary movement) and an up and down (secondary movement). The saddle shape in the center of the ball tends to cradle and support the client laterally, giving more stability. It also encourages a squatting position with support. Use only the 70 cm peanut ball in this position; the other sizes are too small.

- Place client straddling peanut ball
- Only use 70 cm peanut ball to sit on

Note: *See Chapter 8 for detailed information.*

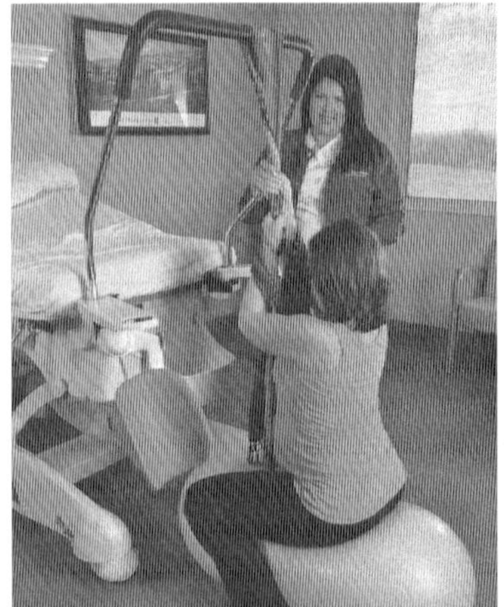

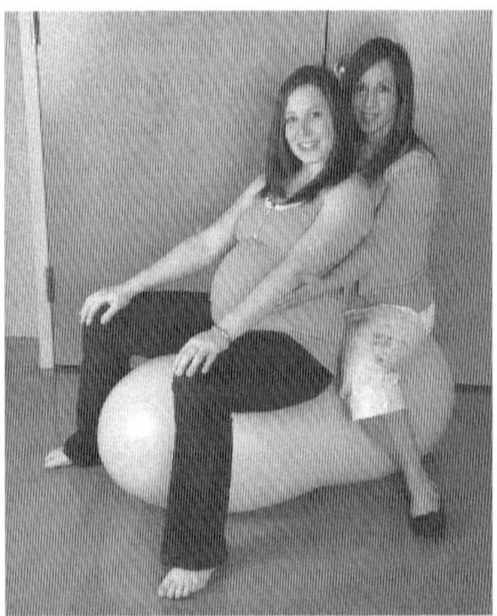

70 cm straddling. *Photos © Premier Birth Tools LLC*

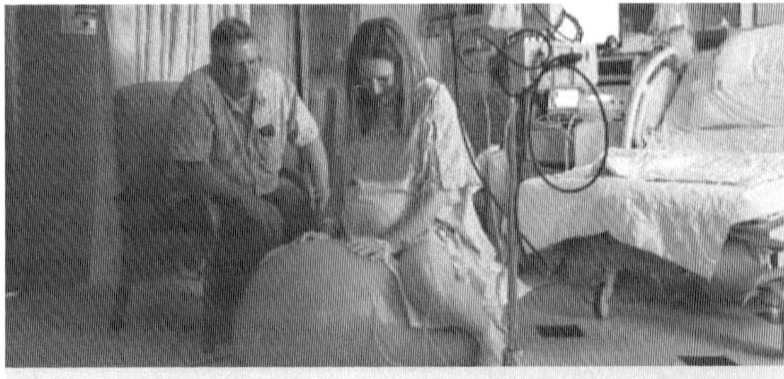

70 cm. *Photo courtesy of Samantha Steen, doula and photographer, CLC*

Pushing with the Peanut Ball

Using a peanut ball during pushing allows the client to rest their legs. This position maintains a wide open posture needed to open the outlet, similar to squatting. The client will hug the peanut ball and pull both legs up to the chest to push. This Tuck Pushing Position is the most common pushing with the peanut ball. We'll review other positions in Chapter 8.

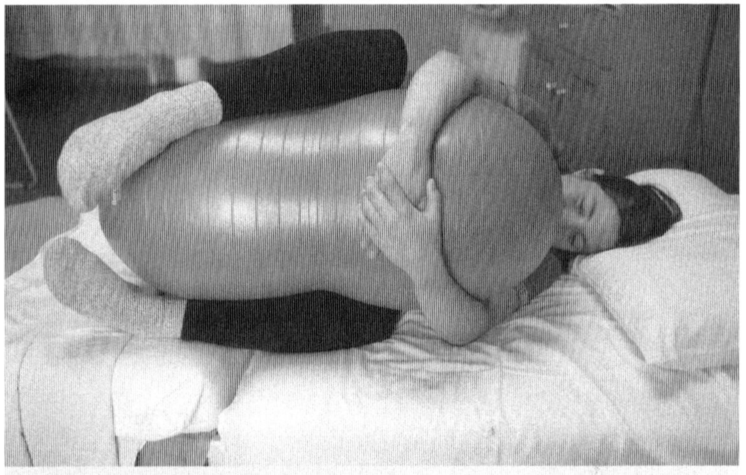

Pushing with the peanut ball in Tuck Position. *Photo © Premier Birth Tools LLC*

> *One of my first experiences when we got the peanut ball was a patient that the physician had made a decision to perform a primary Cesarean Section for failure to progress. He had gone to finish clinic and I suggested that the labor nurse try the peanut ball while we were waiting. We almost ended up with a precipitous nurse delivery in less than an hour!*
>
> Cheryl Fortenberry, nurse, Texas

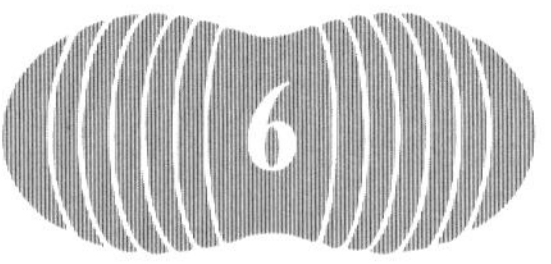

ADVANCED PEANUT BALL POSITIONS

"The peanut ball has changed my life! I have seen it work magic and I want to spread that magic. I want labor nurses to know how to maximize the use of this incredible tool and not just side to side."

—Justine LeDuc, nurse and
Peanut Ball Ambassador, California

IN 2022, THERE ARE NOW more than 50 different peanut ball positions. These new, advanced positions are discussed in future chapters, including:

- Positions to use in relation to where baby is in the pelvis
    - Above the Inlet
    - In the Midpelvis
    - At the Outlet
- Internal and external rotation of femur or thigh bone
- Pushing with peanut ball
- Asymmetrical variations using the peanut ball
- Breech peanut ball tilt
- Fun positions moms invented during labor

In this chapter I have listed additional advanced peanut ball positions not discussed in upcoming chapters.

Squat Rock and Roll

Squat on the peanut ball and gently roll the peanut ball in a rocking side-to-side motion, as the ball would naturally roll. The squatting refers to position, while rocking side-to-side is the motion

1. Place peanut ball between client's legs, while lying on side, with the top leg over the indention
2. Make sure client is turned all the way on their side. Their back should not be flat on the bed
3. Gently roll the peanut ball and rock side to side, as the ball would naturally roll

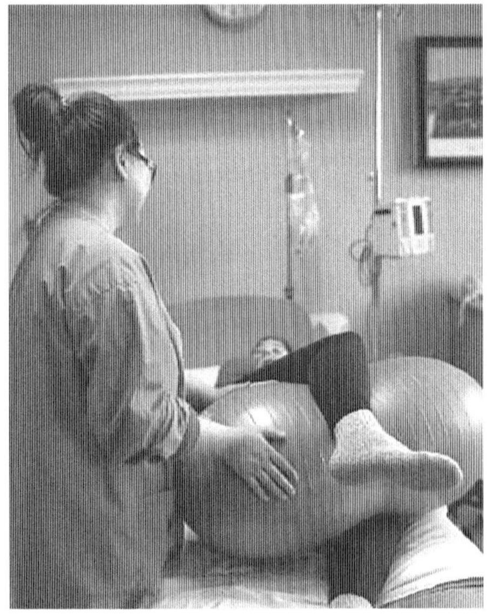

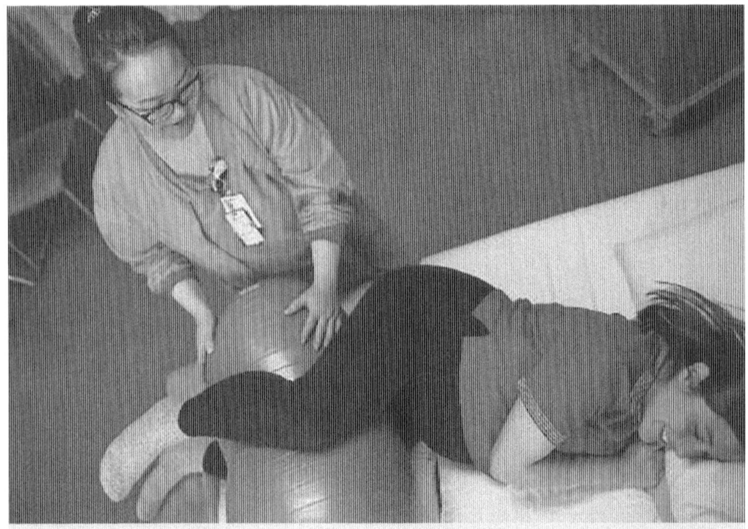

Photos © Premier Birth Tools LLC

SUPPORTED SITTING POSITIONS

Sitting on Peanut Ball Against the Wall

This position allows the client to rest while straddling the peanut ball. The client can sleep when sitting in a corner and possibly resolve an anterior cervical lip by using this position. Pictures show the position that is especially useful during the time when the baby is high above the pelvic inlet. Knees and toes are out, feet are placed out with heels together towards the ball. This causes the desired external rotation of the femur thigh bones.

1. Sitting on the peanut ball in the corner against the wall. Only sit on 70 cm size
2. Place pillows behind the client's low back and support her neck. This enables the client to avoid falling to either side, because the wall is supporting the client
   - An alternative is to place another peanut ball behind the client for greater support depending on client's comfort
   - **Caution:** *Do not place peanut ball next to heater vents while in use on the floor*

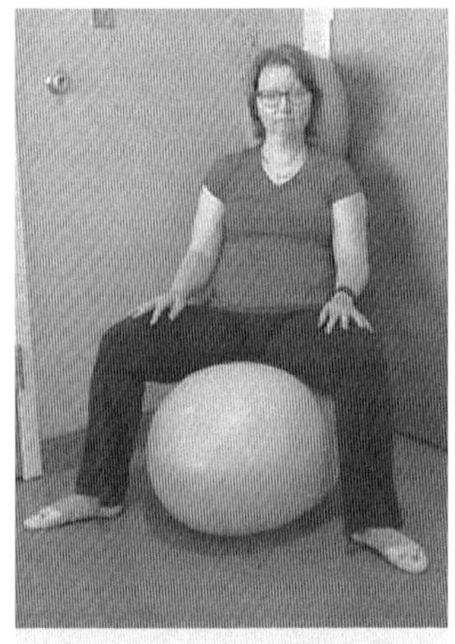

At hospital.
Photo © Premier Birth Tools LLC

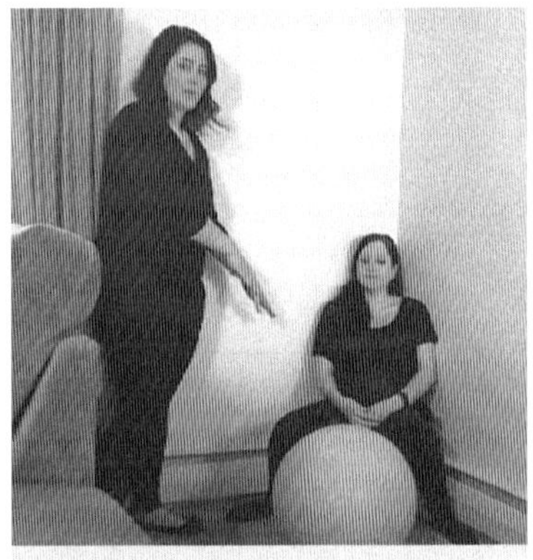

At home. *Photo courtesy of Emma Whitlock*

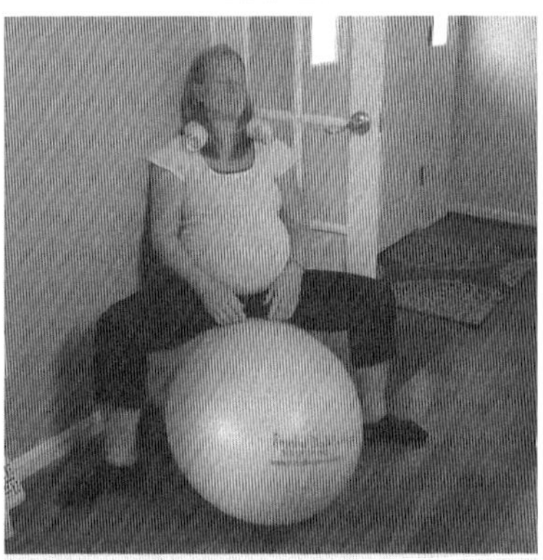

At home. *Photo courtesy of Amy Bookwalter CD*

Sitting on Peanut Ball Supported by Vertical Peanut Ball

By Heidi Duncan CBD (CBI)

This position allows the client to rest while straddling the peanut ball supported by another peanut ball.

1. Sit on 70 cm peanut ball; use only hospital grade to sit on
2. Supported by another peanut ball that is angled vertically toward person to lean forward on for support

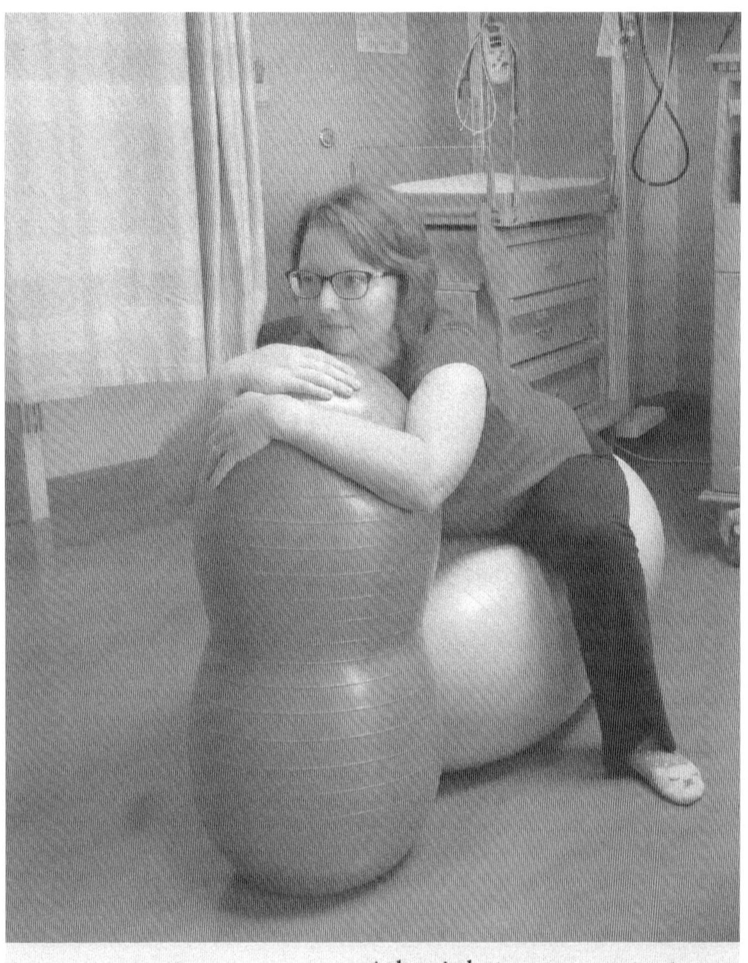

At hospital. *Photo © Premier Birth Tools LLC*

Sitting on Peanut Ball Supported by Peanut Ball

This Forward Leaning Position gives gravitational comfort, eases pressure on the back, and opens the pelvis. The motion and position can facilitate fetal descent.

1. Sit on 70 cm peanut ball; use only hospital thicker grade to sit on
2. Supported by another peanut ball to rest on for support
3. Determine where baby is in pelvis and place knees in correct position

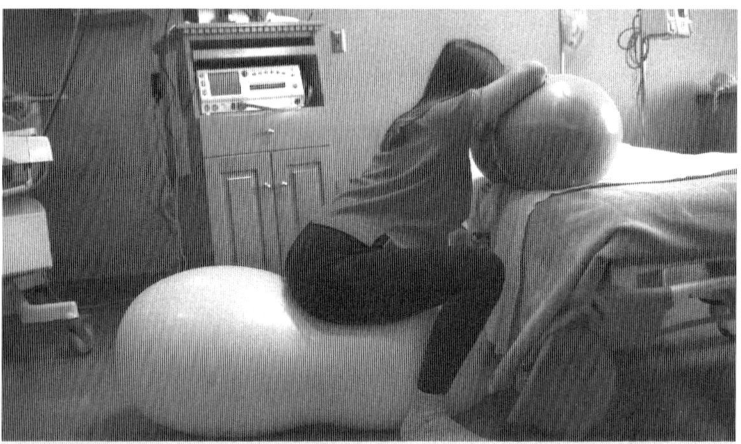

At hospital. *Photo © Premier Birth Tools LLC*

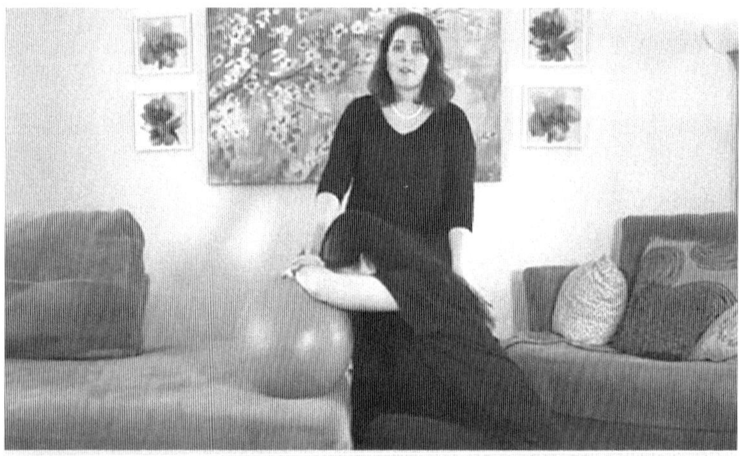

At home. *Photo courtesy of Emma Whitlock*

Resting in Shower

The Peanut Ball is a great tool in the shower and there are many positions that can be used:

1. Resting Straddling peanut ball and Sitting
2. Resting Leaning against wall using peanut ball
3. Sit on peanut ball diagonal or straddling peanut ball
4. Baby above inlet—sit with knees pointing out; baby in middle of pelvis—knees straight; baby in outlet—knees pointing in. *Do not cover the drain with peanut ball.*

Note: *The pictures show a clothed client. When the client's perineal area is uncovered, using a cover on the peanut ball, such as a blue pad (chux), can prevent contamination.*

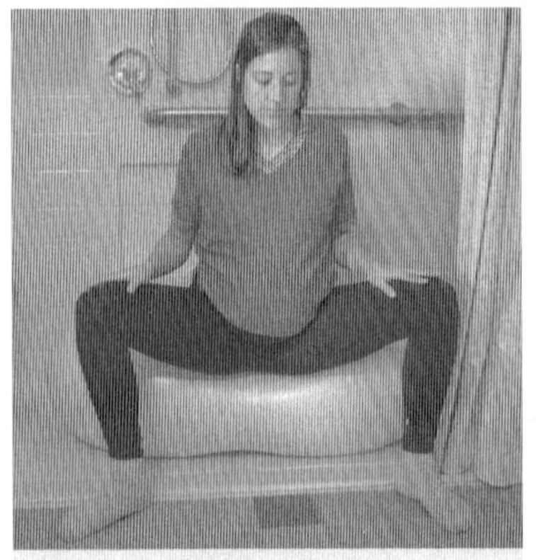

Inlet: knees out

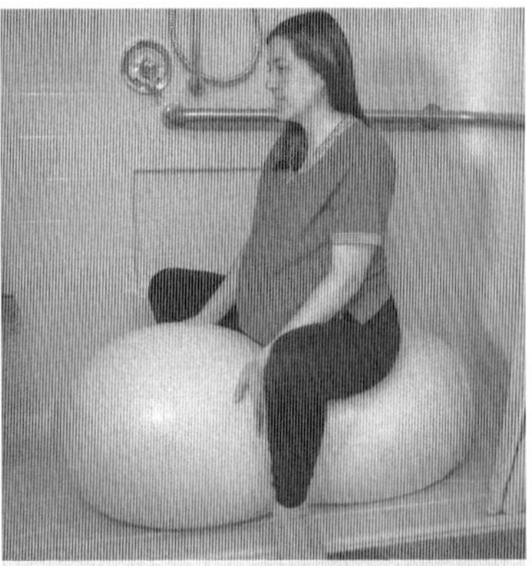

Femurs externally rotated

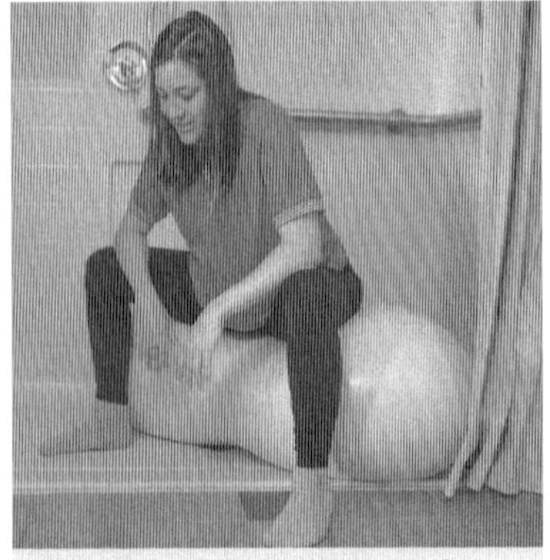

Midpelvis: knees parallel

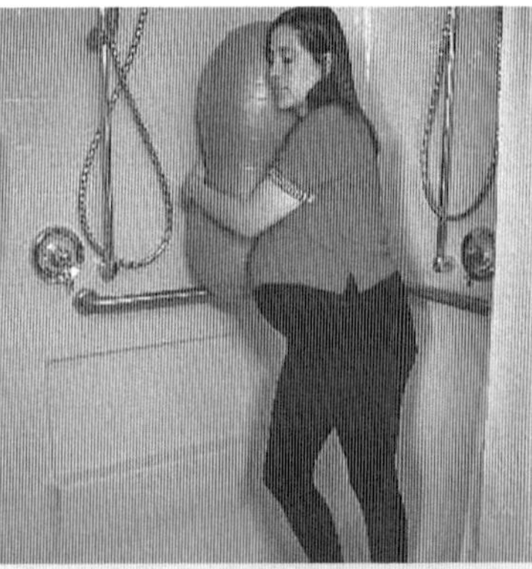

Midpelvis: knees neutral

> *I'm passionate about peanut ball usage, and really want to integrate use of the larger ball for more movement in labor and shower. I bring them to almost every birth.*
>
> Heather McCullough, midwife, Illinois

Resting in Tub

The peanut ball can be used to help a client rest in the tub. A client can sit on the peanut ball or kneel in the tub, leaning forward on the peanut ball, which is angled away. Rebekah Porter states, "Peanut balls are traditionally used landside, but they can also be very useful in the tub. Give it to the mom to lean on while laboring in the tub. After tub use, remember to clean the ball thoroughly and let dry."

1. Sit on 70 cm peanut ball; use only hospital grade to sit on
2. Supported by another peanut ball to rest on for support

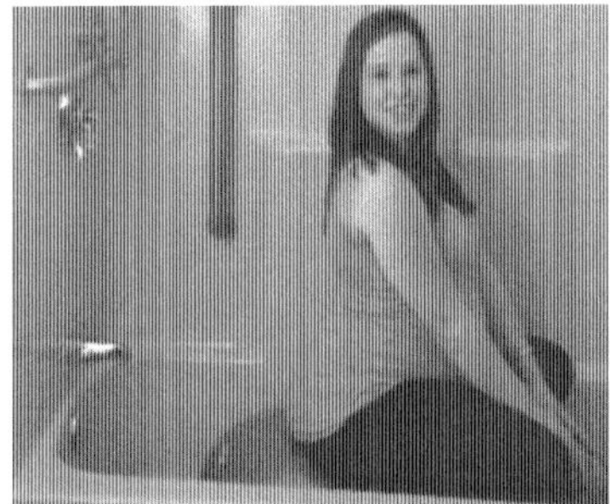

Photo © Premier Birth Tools LLC

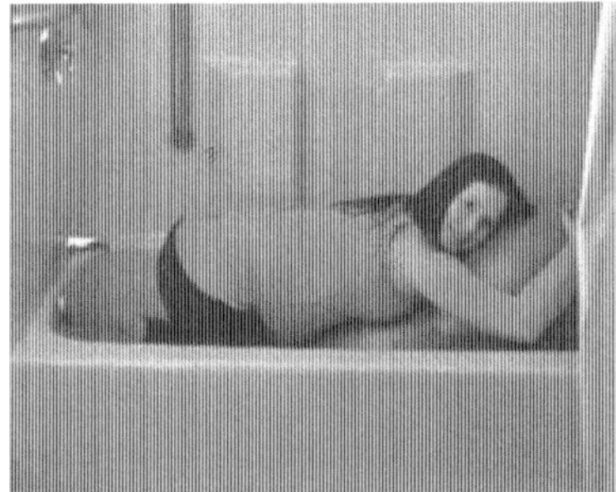

Photo © Premier Birth Tools LLC

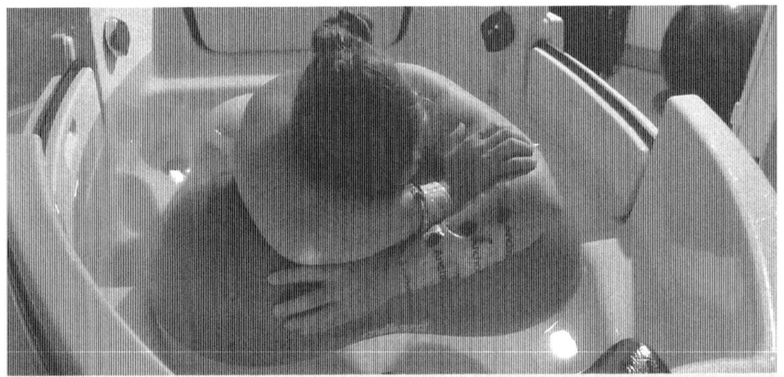

Photo courtesy of Rebekah Porter, Blissful Birthing

I love to use the peanut ball to not only help with baby position, but it is also useful to make mom more comfortable.

Rebekah Porter, doula and Peanut Ball Ambassador, Tennessee

Hands and Knees, Kneeling and Straddling

This position requires two peanut balls. Place the client on their hands and knees. Have them straddle one peanut ball and lean forward onto a smaller peanut ball. Be aware that in this position the back-end of the peanut ball may want to pop up. To avoid this, keep a hand pressing down towards the bed on the back-end of the ball. You can also use a sheet to tie that end of the peanut ball to the bed.

1. Place client on hands and knees and lower the bottom of the bed
2. Have client lean forward onto a smaller peanut ball
3. Straddle peanut ball; use only hospital grade to sit on

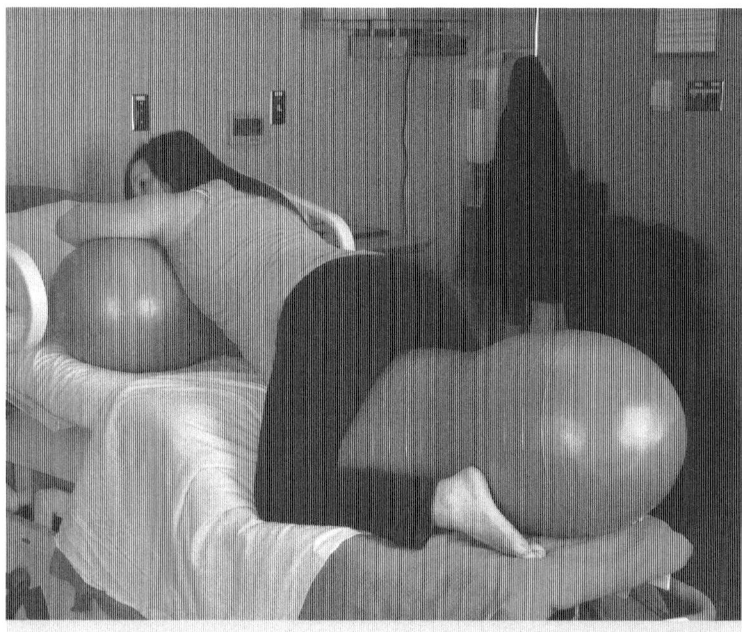

Photo © Premier Birth Tools LLC

Using a Rebozo with a Client

Honor the Culture by being Properly Trained

Rebozo use can facilitate peanut ball positions (pictured on the following page). The Rebozo is a long, rectangular cloth that has been used by various people groups in several countries over many generations. Rebozos can help facilitate several peanut ball positions, but it is important to have proper training for their use to honor the cultures traditionally using this tool, and to avoid cultural appropriatation (using items from a culture that is not our own.) This protects the client's safety and honors both the culture of the Rebozo and those midwives who have been gracious to pass down its traditional use. We are all guardians of the ancestral midwife practices. Our responsibility is to embrace their wisdom, give honor and respect to its use, and thus have their "blessing."

I have studied under Gina Kirby, Debra Pascali, Polly Perez, and Marlita Camacho. Also, I want to honor Guadalupe Trueba, Doña Irene Sotelo, and Naolí Vinaver, who showed me correct uses of the Rebozo at a midwifery conference. I was given permission to use this picture and others in this book by an indigenous person, who was at this demonstration.

Learn More

Visit Naolí Vinave's website to learn more about how to use a Rebozo in her workshops: naolivinaver.com

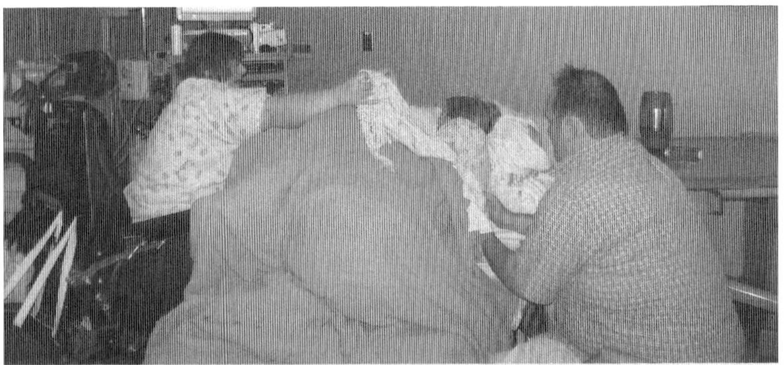

Cheri with client, using rebozo and peanut ball. *Photo © Premier Birth Tools LLC*

Note: *You should only use the Rebozo if you've received proper training. Use a sheet if not properly trained.*

Over the Door or Squat Bar

A client may use a sheet or Rebozo over the door or squat bar for more stability.

1. Sit on 70 cm peanut ball; use only hospital grade to sit on
2. Use a sheet or Rebozo over the door or squat bar
3. Tie a knot in the sheet or Rebozo, toss knot over the door and shut the door so the sheet or Rebozo will not pull through
4. Determine where baby is in pelvis and place knees in correct position discussed in later chapter

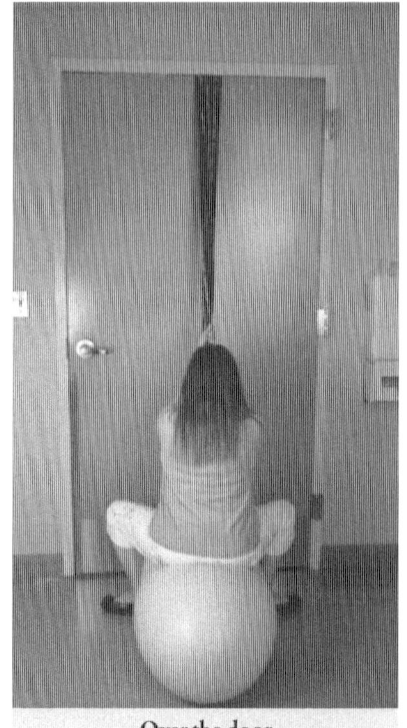

Over the door

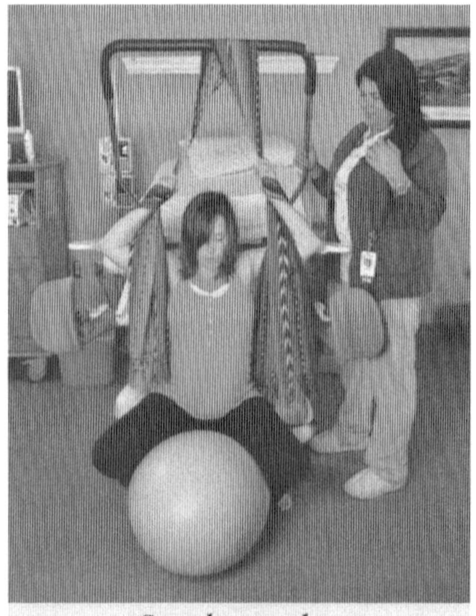

Over the squat bar

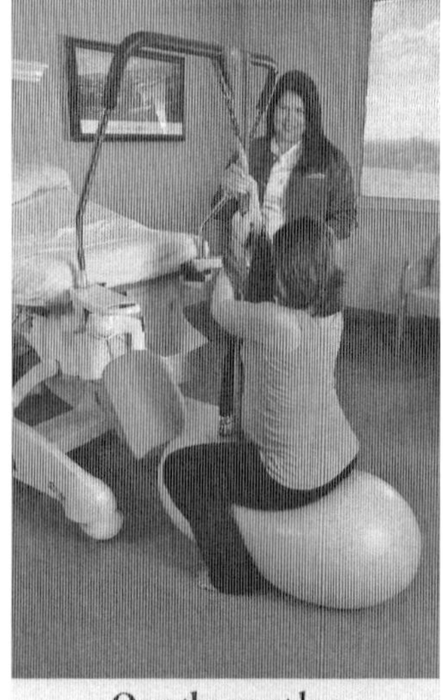

Over the squat bar

Lotus

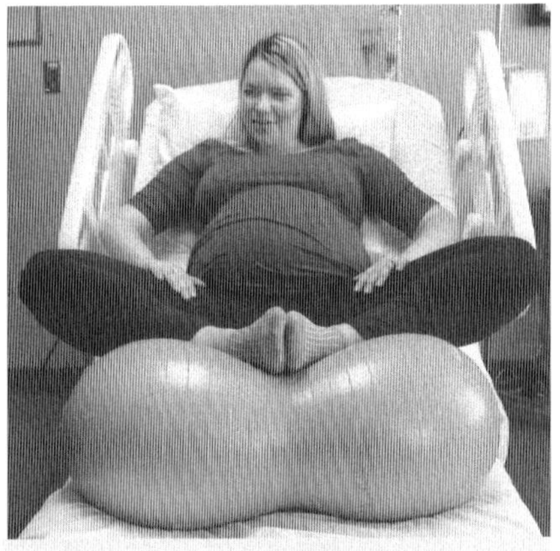

Lotus Position. *Photo © Premier Birth Tools LLC*

This position is typically used for clients with epidurals, as it helps them to labor down if the baby is high in the pelvis. Do not use if the station is -1 or below. The position opens the top of the pelvis and inlet, and closes the bottom. If the legs are heavy, due to the epidural, lower the foot of the bed and place feet on top of the ball. The bed can then be raised to elevate the ball to the desired height. Nikki Zerfas states, "This can be extreme for some clients without flexibility. If they have an epidural, they may not feel the over-stretching. Having just one leg bent in a sort of 'half-lotus' and the other leg extended is another position to offer clients, who have chosen an epidural prior to engagement." See Chapter 8 for Semi-Sitting Lunge Position and more details.

1. Head of bed slightly up. Client is semi-reclined in bed
2. Lower the foot of the bed and place feet on top of the ball. The bed can then be raised to elevate the ball to the desired height

> *My favorite method is to put a patient in the Texas Roll with a peanut ball when she is in active labor. Typically, the baby will spin and descend. They progress very quickly and rarely have to push. I've used it multiple times. We also have a very small peanut ball that I am learning to use. We use it to put the heel higher than the patient's knee, which seems to facilitate descent from a minus station to a 0 or lower.*
>
> Paula Kivett, nurse, Indiana

I can't count the number of times I have come on shift and started using the peanut ball, and moving my patient and quickly getting my patient complete and delivered after they have laid in the same position all day.

Lindsay Randolph nurse, Peanut Ball Ambassador, Missouri

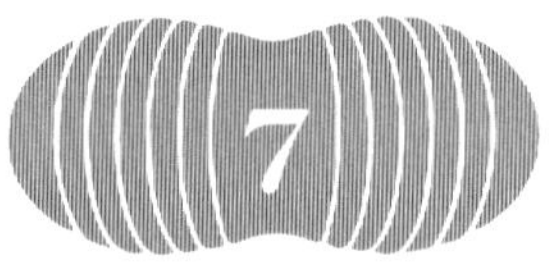

POSITIONS FOR USE IN RELATION TO BABY'S LOCATION IN PELVIS

"We love the peanut balls. We believe they help with descent and delivery and give laboring patients more options."

—Nurses at Family Birthplace, University of Maryland Upper Chesapeake Medical Center in Bel Air, Maryland

THE BABY'S POSITION in the pelvis is an important factor when choosing a peanut ball position. In this chapter, I will share location specifics and basic peanut balls positions for each. Advanced positions will be described for each location in following chapters.

PLACE THE KNEES CORRECTLY

In these positions, placement of the knees is more helpful to observe than the feet. Feet can go in any direction, but the knees are specific and directly connect to the pelvis. Specific knee placement is outlined in following chapters.

Recently, a nurse from Mississippi called and asked me to explain how to place the knees on the peanut ball. The nurse said, "I have a patient in labor, who has previously spoken to you on the phone; I need to understand what she is trying to tell me." I told the nurse, "Here is the quick guide to remember:

First, sit in your chair placing your heels together and knees out; this is if the baby is above the inlet -4, -3, -2 station.

Second, sit straight in your chair with knees pointing forward; this is if the baby is in the midpelvis at a 0 station.

Third, put your knees and toes together; this is if the baby is visible and below the outlet."

As I was talking, I could hear on the other end, "Wow! That makes total sense! I get it now. Thank you!" In one minute, I taught this nurse something that she will always remember while using peanut balls in labor.

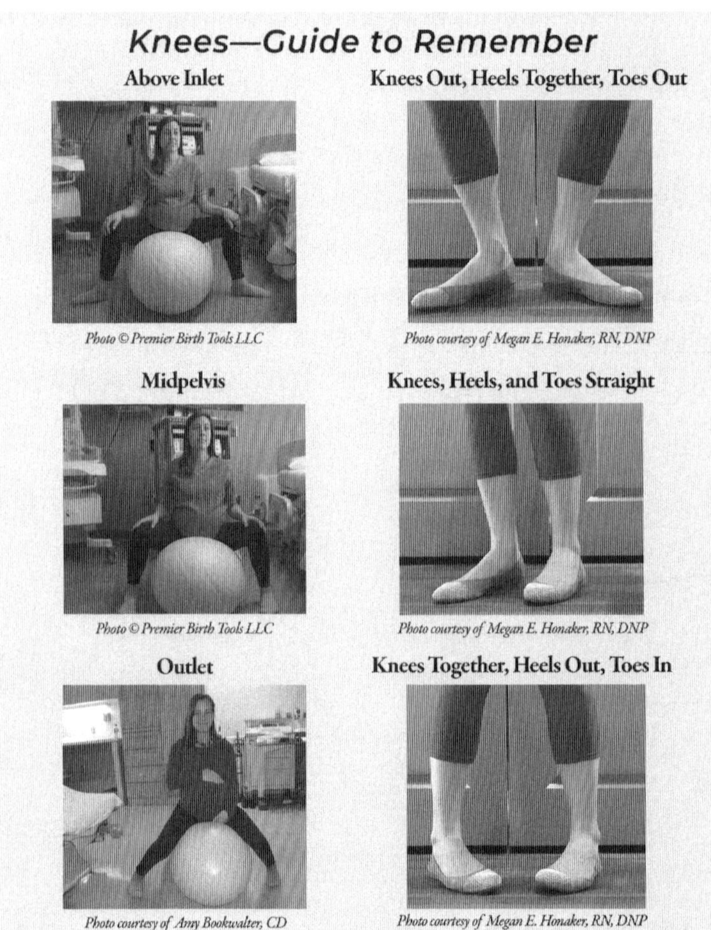

Photo © Premier Birth Tools LLC

Photo courtesy of Megan E. Honaker, RN, DNP

Photo © Premier Birth Tools LLC

Photo courtesy of Megan E. Honaker, RN, DNP

Photo courtesy of Amy Bookwalter, CD

Photo courtesy of Megan E. Honaker, RN, DNP

THE BABY'S POSITION IN THE PELVIS

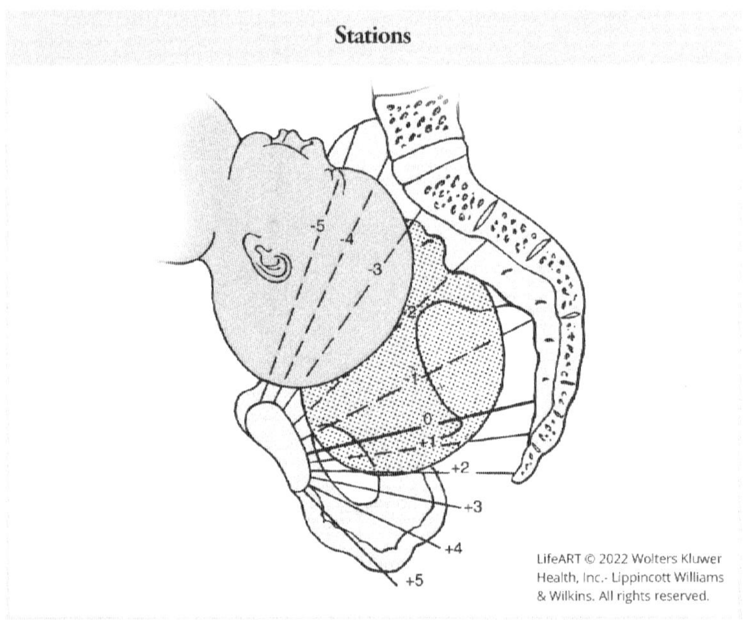

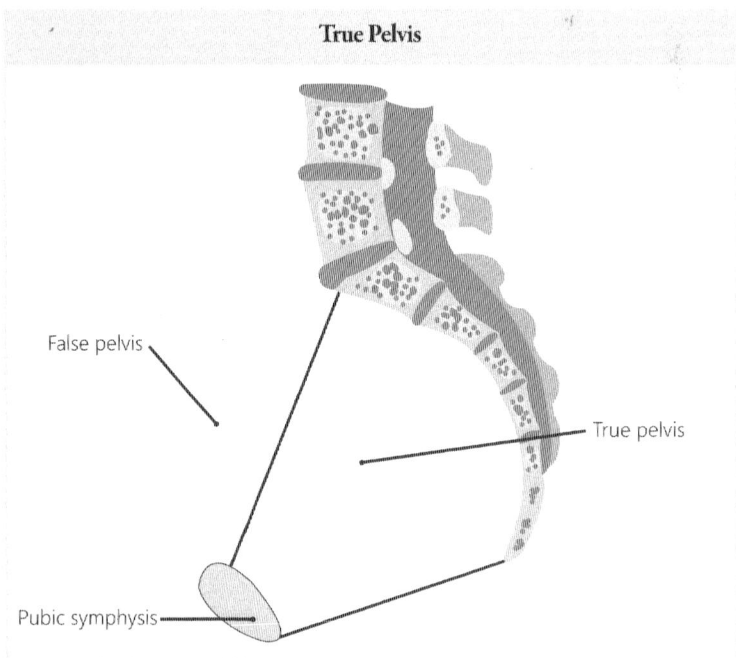

Above the Inlet

- Baby is high in the pelvis and not dropped down
- Client will feel the baby up under the rib cage and it is hard to breathe
- -4, -3 or -2 station or higher
- Inlet is usually wider from side to side and narrower from front to back
- Open inlet, rotating femur thigh bone by external rotation; widen knees and posterior pelvic tilt by flattening low back
- Movement more forward and backwards in rocking; tuck buttocks, spread knees apart
- Position peanut ball with clients knees out, heels together, and feet pointing out in opposite directions

Note: *See Chapter 8 for detailed information and positions for the inlet.*

Example of Inlet Postion: *Semi-Sitting Lunge*

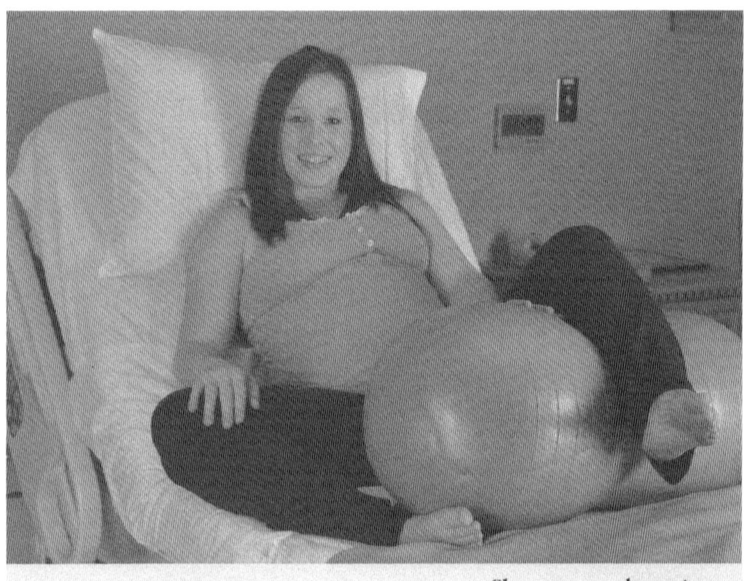

Shows external rotation.

Photo © Premier Birth Tools LLC

Note: *See Chapter 8 for detailed information about this position.*

Midpelvis

- Baby is engaged
- -1,0, +1 station
- Widest part at diagonal diameter
- Opens front to back—midpelvis
- Movement includes sideways, diagonal, and uneven hip, including lunges and peanut ball movements. Create a rotation in pelvis that opens diagonally; sideways movements open pelvis floor side to side to allow rotation and descent
- Position peanut ball between client's legs, pointing knees straight forward, parallel, and neutral

Note: *See Chapter 9 for detailed information and positions for midpelvis.*

Example of Midpelvis Postion: *Side-Lying Parallel Position*

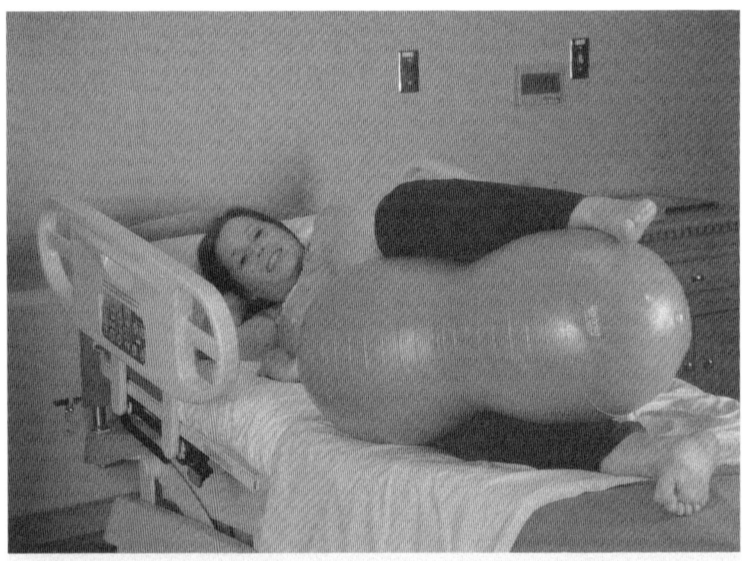

Shows parallel and neutral position.

Photo courtesy of Amy Emerson, RN, Doula for Birth

Note: *See Chapter 9 for detailed information about this position.*

Outlet

- Baby is low in the pelvis and client is ready to push
- +2, +3 station or lower—you can see the baby
- Most space is front to back—increase with movement of sacrum and coccyx (tailbone) as opening is outward movement of the sacrum
- Open "outlet" side to side, by rotating femur or thigh bone to internal rotation, causing the ischial tuberosities (sitz bones) to move farther apart
- Position peanut ball between client's ankles with knees together, heels out, and toes pointing toward each other

Note: *See Chapter 10 for detailed information positions for the Outlet.*

Example of Outlet Postion: *Knees Together, Heels Out*

Popularized in the U.S. by Spinning Babies® Approved Trainers

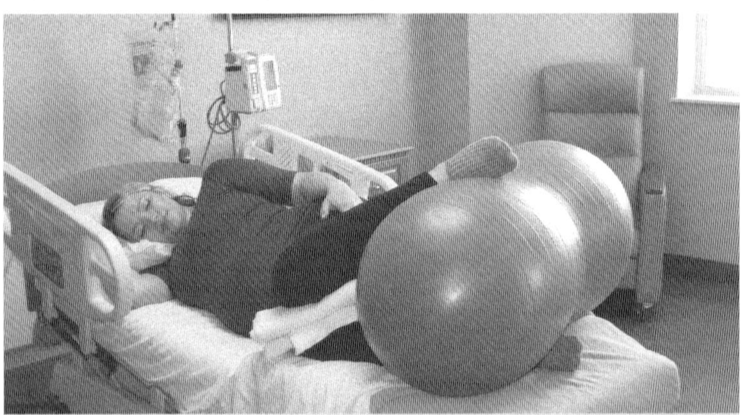

Shows internal rotation. Place peanut ball between ankles and towel between knees. *Photo © Premier Birth Tools LLC*

Note: *See Chapter 10 for detailed information about this position.*

Learn More

For more information on levels of the pelvis, visit Spinning Babies® by Gail Tully, CPM (Spinning Babies® 2021): spinningbabies.com/solutions-for-dystocia-in-the-levels-of-the-pelvis

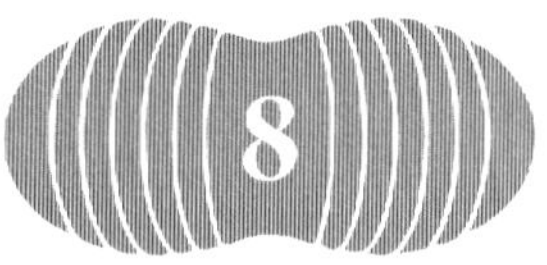

POSITIONS FOR ABOVE THE INLET

"I have seen the peanut ball help to open a mom up to get baby's head more engaged."

—Maureen Vuraich, nurse, Ohio

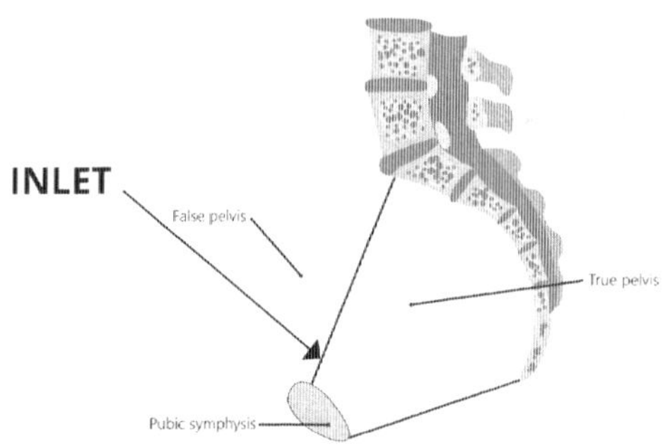

INLET TOP OF PELVIS

External rotation makes room for baby to come in to the pelvis

Inlet = Baby In
External rotation of femur thigh bones = Inlet = Get baby In
External opens Top of pelvis
Knees pointing Outward = Knees Out
Heels together and toes pointing out in opposite directions
Knees Pointing Outward—Opens Inlet Top of pelvis

POSITIONS FOR ABOVE THE INLET

The inlet is located at the top of the pelvis. When the baby is above the inlet, it is high, not engaged, and the brim may need to be opened. To open the inlet, externally rotate the femur or thigh bone by opening the knees wide and using posterior pelvic tilt. Flatten the lower back and tilt the pelvis forward. Rock forwards and backwards, keeping the buttocks tucked and the knees spread. Use this position when the baby is high in the pelvis and not dropped down -4,-3, or -2 station or higher.

Knee Position: *When using inlet positions it is important that knees are pointing outward with external rotation of femur or thigh bone and the toes in opposite positions.*

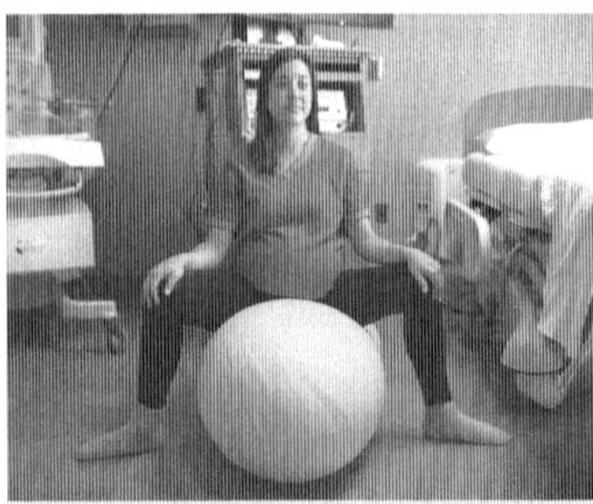

Knees pointing outward, above the inlet, opens top pelvis. *Photo © Premier Birth Tools LLC*

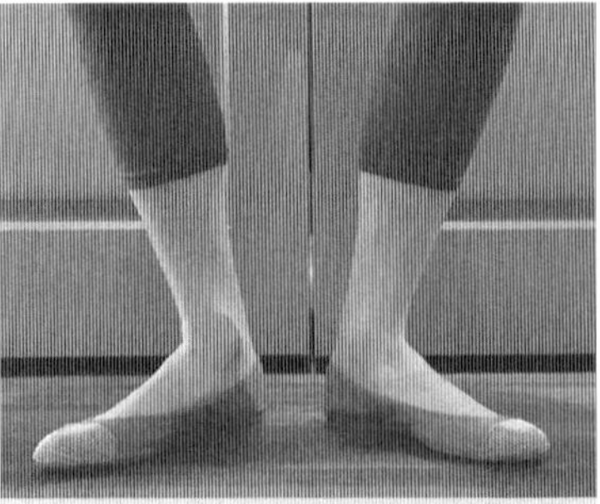

Heels together, pointing in opposite directions. *Photo courtesy of Megan E. Honaker, RN, DNP*

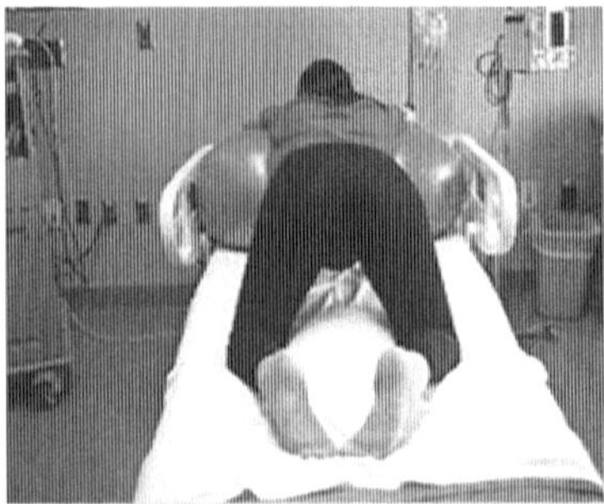

Inlet on peanut ball. Knees pointing out, external rotation of femur bones opening top of pelvis. *Photo © Premier Birth Tools LLC*

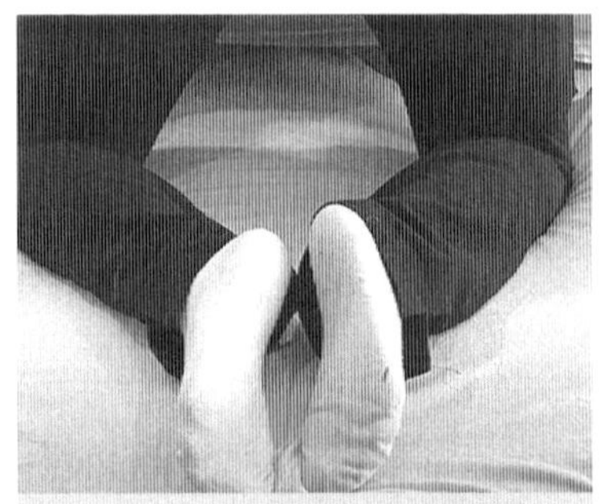

External rotation of femur or thigh bone. *Photo courtesy of Megan E. Honaker, RN, DNP*

Hands and Knees

Resting on the peanut ball provides comfort and ensures the client is hanging the baby so it can turn to the optimal position, especially if occiput posterior or asynclitic. Leaning forward will provide some gravity advantage and align the baby with the pelvis. This position will aid in opening the inlet, as well as in reducing an anterior cervical lip.

On hands and knees, the rotation of the femur can change from external, to neutral, to internal by rotating the feet. *Follow the knees.* If the knee is pointing *in*, towards the other knee, that makes for internal rotation. If the knee is pointing *out*, away from the other knee, that leg is doing external rotation.

1. Place client on hands and knees and lower bottom of the bed
2. Have client lean over the peanut ball
3. On hands and knees, with knees wide apart pointing out and feet close together—external rotation of femur or thigh bone
4. On hands and knees with knees wide apart, external rotation of femurs happens when feet are close together. *To view internal rotation, see picture on page 115.*
5. In kneeling position, external rotation—knees are wide and feet are close. Internal rotation—feet are wide apart and knees are turned inward.

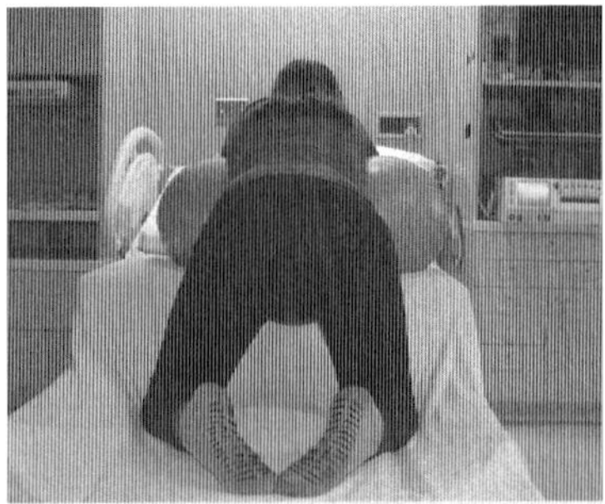

In hospital. External rotation of femur or thigh bone, knees out.

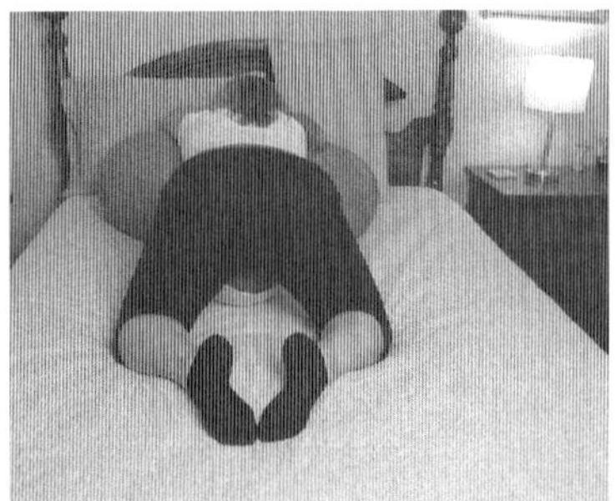

At home. External rotation of femur or thigh bone, knees out.

Photos courtesy of Amt Bookwalter, CD

Flying Cowgirl Position

By Gail Tully, CPM, Spinning Babies®

This position is used to help open the inlet. The reason this works is because the quadriceps femur thigh muscle attaches at the front of the pelvis to the knee. The Flying Cowgirl Position helps the pelvis open toward the front. It also helps stretch the psoas to help engagement and open the brim. The back is in a straight line.

1. Place peanut ball between client's knees, causing external rotation of femur or thigh bone, which opens inlet more side to side
2. With pubic bone forward, push the hips forward until they lock as the client kicks the legs backwards. This pushes the pelvis in a posterior pelvic tilt, which opens the pelvis more front to back. *Be sure to have client's femur or thigh bone straight down from her body, with no bend in her hip, and her knees bent as far as she is able to bend them backwards.*
3. Knees in and ankles out

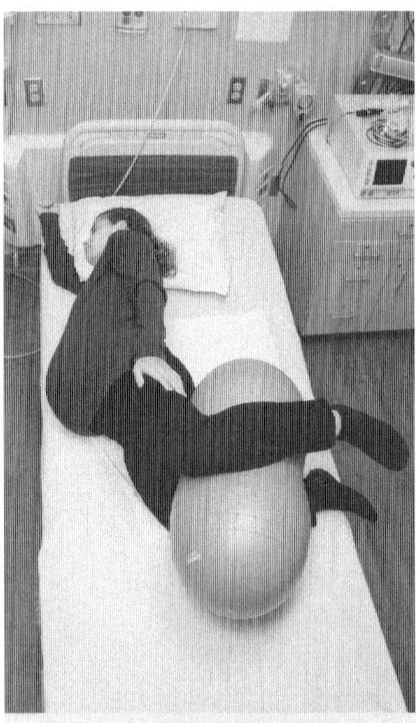

Photo courtesy of Amy Bookwalter, CD

Nikki Zerfas, RN, SpBT, states, "A tip for making this position more comfortable and balanced, is to lower the foot of the bed . . . by 2–3 inches—just a little! This balances the angles in both hips and centers the ball between the legs."

Caution: *This position makes an extreme angle from the spine to the pubic bone. Back injury may make spine worse. Arching puts pressure on discs.*

The key to this position is ensuring the angle between the belly and the femur or thigh bone is as open as possible. Make sure the heels are together and the knees are pointing outward. *Note that the tendency with this position is for the client to gradually relax and pull their knees forward into a plain side-lying posture.* Having back support can keep their hips pushed forward into proper alignment. Flying Cowgirl is a variation for Side-Lying Position instead of being supine in the Walcher Position.

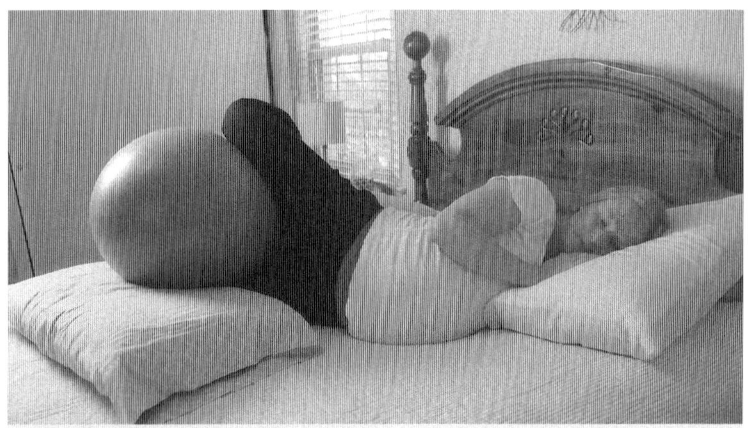

At home, Flying Cowgirl with knees bent back. Helps baby drop into pelvis.
Photo courtesy of Amy Bookwalter, CD

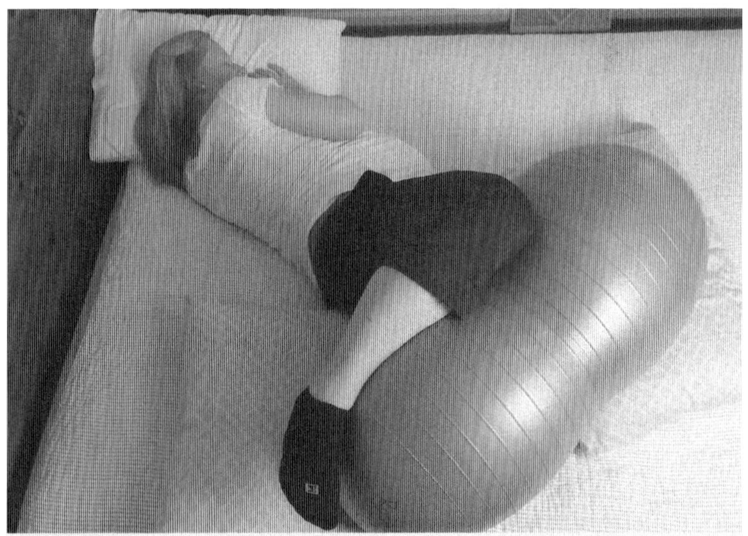

Correct alignment: back straight with feet barely hanging off.
Photo courtesy of Amy Bookwalter, CD

Nulliparous, 5–6 hours on 7–8 cm dilated, high caput, with epidural on the maximum of oxytocin. She was up for a Cesarean. Then my shift started; did the peanut ball both sides (Flying Cowgirl) for 45 minutes to open the inlet. Result: fully dilated and urge to push. Switched to peanut ball between under legs to open the outlet, and 15 minutes later baby was born!

Marloes Faber, midwife and Peanut Ball Ambassador, The Netherlands

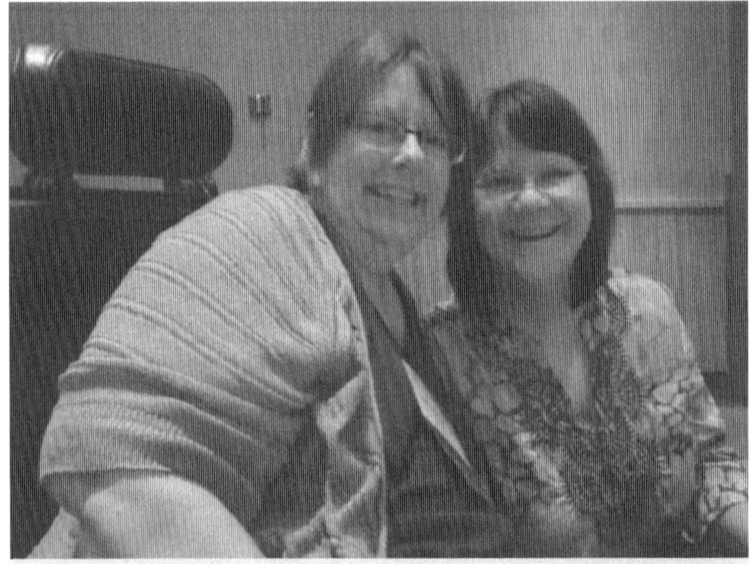

Cheri Grant (left) and Gail Tully of Spinning Babies® (right).

Fun Fact

How the "Flying Cowgirl" Position was Created

By Cheri Grant, RN

This position was created at the 2014 LAMAZE/DONA conference after my presentation, discussing new peanut ball positions with Gail Tully, CPM, from Spinning Babies®. Gail made a drawing of this position and said it looked like someone riding a bronco. Since I'm from Oklahoma, we decided to call it the "Flying Cowgirl."

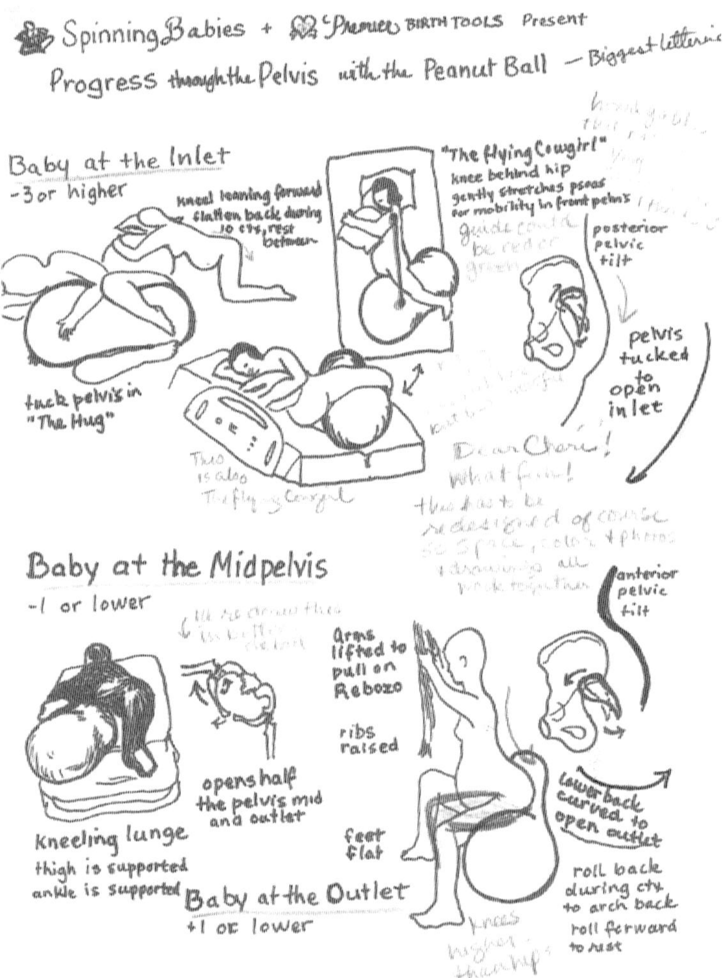

Drawing of new peanut ball positions.

©Spinning Babies® & Premier Birth Tools LLC

Learn More

Gail Tully, CPM, from Spinning Babies® has excellent information regarding Inlet, Midpelvis, and Outlet of progression through the pelvis. Gail has a unique approach to birth through her three principles of Spinning Babies®: release with Balance, Gravity, and Movement℠ (Spinning Babies, 2021). To learn more visit: spinningbabies.com.

Standing Walchers

This position is used to help open the inlet. Back is in a straight line; client's knees are out; heels pointing inward and toes pointing outwards. This is a plie' standing and leaning backwards over the peanut ball.

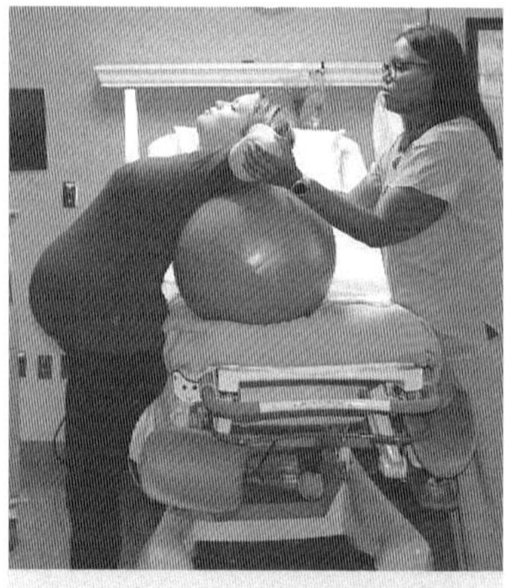

Photo © Premier Birth Tools LLC

- Standing, leaning backwards over peanut ball
- Knees out, feet with heels pointing inward and toes pointing outwards
- Arch bend opens the brim

I received a patient that was 'arrested descent' at -1 station, so I used the peanut ball to position my patient to Flying Cowgirl and then to Walchers to assist with fetal descent. Patient delivered vaginally approximately one hour later.

Onika Davis, nurse, California

Exaggerated

One nurse exaggerated the Flying Cowgirl by having the client reach back and grab her feet like a yoga pose. This could hurt client's quad and spine if they are not limber. If the client is a yogini (regular and long-term yoga practitioner) they likely wouldn't mind this.

- Start with a straight line from shoulder to knee, then exaggerate the pelvis forward even more. Butt is touching peanut ball
- Walchers refers to the upperback and shoulders leaning or arching backward, thus arching the midback and making the abdomen very prominent in front
- Walcher is a German doctor who practiced in the late 1800s and whose name is associated with a midwife technique, first published in the 1500s, that has been proven to open the inlet.

The Flying Cowgirl is a variation for Side Lying instead of being supine on the very edge of the bed.

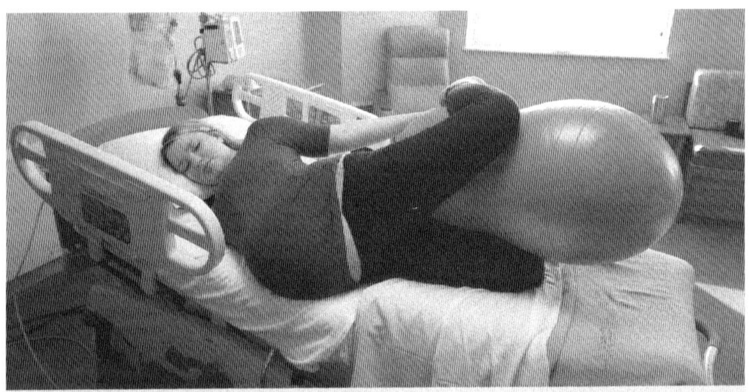

Photo © Premier Birth Tools LLC

Caution: *Epiduralized client may not recognize if they are over-stretching and this could lead to injuries or pain after the epidural is gone. This position makes an extreme angle from the spine to the pubic bone. Back injury may make spine worse. Arching puts pressure on discs.*

A friend called me during her labor of her second baby and said her OB was talking Cesarean Section, as she had not progressed past 4 cm and -2 for 12+ hours. She had been lying flat in bed (post epidural) for 6 of those 12 hours. She asked me to help. I asked for a peanut ball for repositioning and better pelvic opening. The nurse brought in a tiny, half deflated peanut ball and said she didn't know what to do with it. I asked if they had a bigger size (based off the mom's height) and the ability to inflate it properly. First, I put the mom in Flying Cowgirl for several contractions and then moved her into Semi-Sitting Lunge Position alternating legs every 20-30 minutes with the peanut ball. The baby was born less than 2 hours after I showed up and got the mom "moving" . . . everyone was thrilled!"

Aubrey Williams, doula and Peanut Ball Ambassador, Indiana

Kneeling Walchers

By Heidi Duncan CBD (CBI)

Authorized Peanut Ball Trainer, Evidence Based Birth® Instructor, Expecting New Life Birth Services

The ball is against the midback, forcing the back to arch and the hips to push forward. The smaller ball behind the hips helps press the hips forward. While this doesn't have the gravity-neutral advantage of the original Walchers position, it aims to create a similar posture. This position could also be used with abdominal lift for a "lift and tuck" variation.

- Peanut ball is against the midback, forcing the back to arch
- Place smaller ball behind the hips to help press the hips forward
- Can be used with abdominal lift for a "lift and tuck" variation

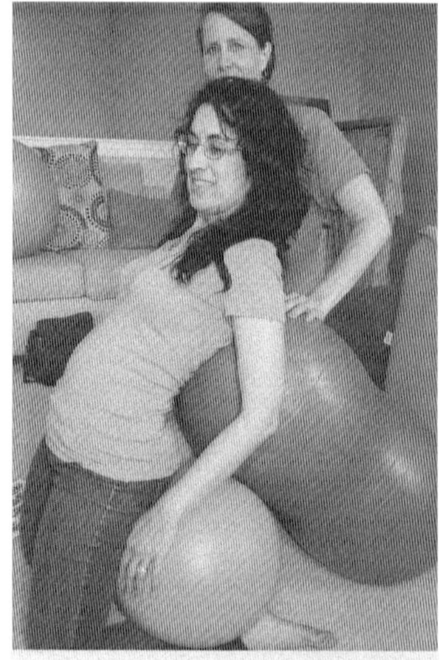

Photo courtesy of Heidi Duncan, CBD (CBI), Expecting New Life

Tailor Walchers

Opens the top of the pelvis to help baby drop in during contraction.

- Feet together, tailor sitting, arching back Walchers over peanut ball with posterior pelvic tilt
- Client uses the peanut ball for better arch. Place towel under buttocks for better tilt
- Alternative is Froggie Walcher's Position (no peanut ball). It opens the top of the pelvis to help baby drop in during contractions. Froggie Walcher, from Alaskan Midwives, does not use the peanut ball. Put a roll under client's hips. Knees should drop lower than hips.

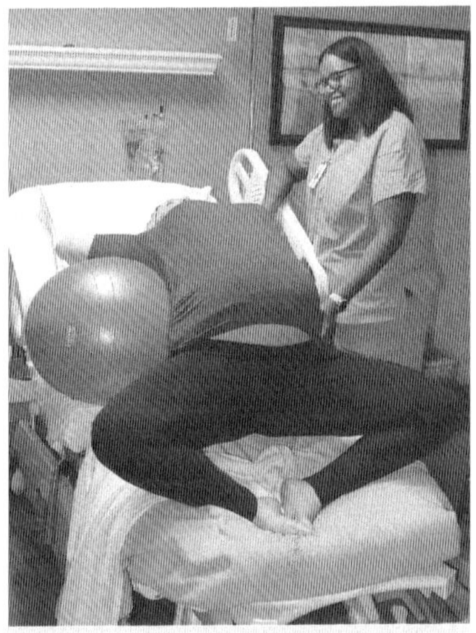
Photo © Premier Birth Tools LLC

Gail Tully CPM, Spinning Babies®, discusses Froggie Walcher on her website and her new book: *Changing Birth on Earth: A Midwife and Nurse's Guide to Using Physiology to Avoid Another Unnecessary Cesarean* (Tully, 2020).

Supported Knee Chest

By Penny Simkin, PT

This position is for use with a -4 or -3 station and will help back baby out of the pelvic brim to start again in better position.

- On hands and knees, lower chest to floor or bed so buttocks are higher than chest
- Use a peanut ball for support if tired and maintain position
- Pelvis is tucked to open the inlet
- Knee-Chest opens the angle of the symphysis
- Knees far apart will open the pelvic inlet bigger at the top in the front-to-back
- Peanut ball is used to support client in this position
- May reduce anterior lip or swollen cervix

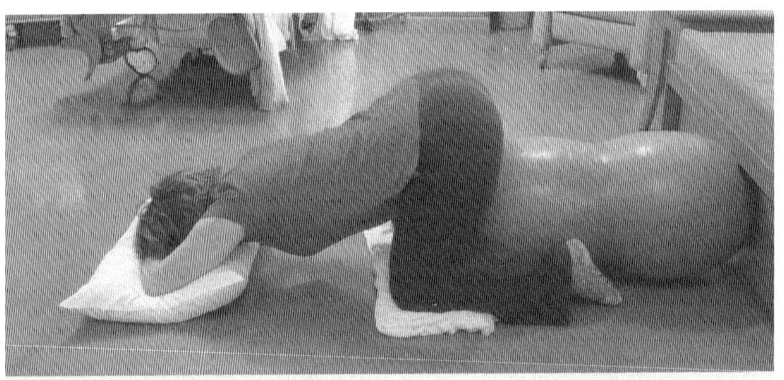
Photo © Premier Birth Tools LLC

Side-Lying Lunge

This position encourages the baby to move up and reposition its head, tuck its chin, and come back down. This position will slightly torque the client's pelvis, close the bottom of the outlet, and will open the inlet making more or less room in that area of the pelvis. This position has several different names: Texas Roll, Runners, Exaggerated Sims, Semi-Prone, and more.

- This position is the same as lunging
- The bottom leg is straight. The top leg is bent 90-degrees with the foot over and in front of the peanut ball while lying on side. Caution, if knee is tipped down then it is a neutral position
- The upper body needs to rotate so the chest is facing down on the bed, like trying to sleep on their stomach
- Laying with the baby's back toward the ceiling will help gravity to turn the baby

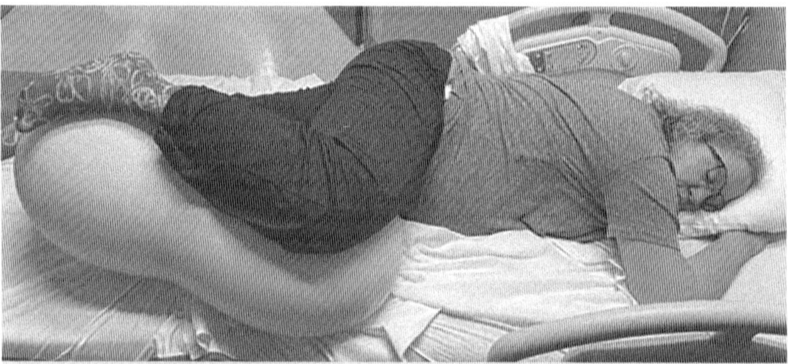

Photo courtesy of Amy Emerson, RN, Doula for Birth

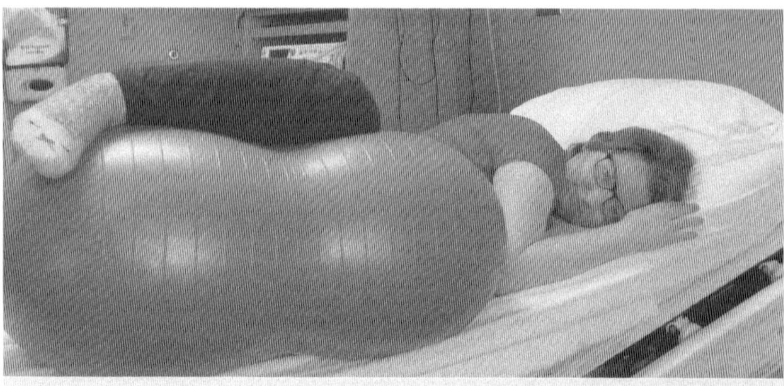

This ball is too big. *Photo © Premier Birth Tools LLC*

> *The peanut ball helped a client avoid a Cesarean after 28 hours of labor, with a swollen and stalled cervix.*
>
> Heather Viers, doula, Florida

Semi-Sitting Lunge

In Semi-Sitting Lunge, the client is semi-reclined on the bed with one leg over the ball at the knee, and the other leg on the bed, like a butterfly. This position encourages descent and may increase the inlet and descent if knees are out. It also promotes dilation, as the head is more applied to the cervix in an upright position. Allowing the client to lunge will open more on one side of pelvis. Do not have the client sitting straight up or it may cause too much pressure on the sacrum and coccyx.

- One leg over the peanut ball, lying in the dip in the middle of the peanut ball
- Leg is over peanut ball
- Other leg is in the Tailor Position and bent
- Heels together ,toes pointing out in opposite directions
- External rotation of femur or thigh bone, knees out

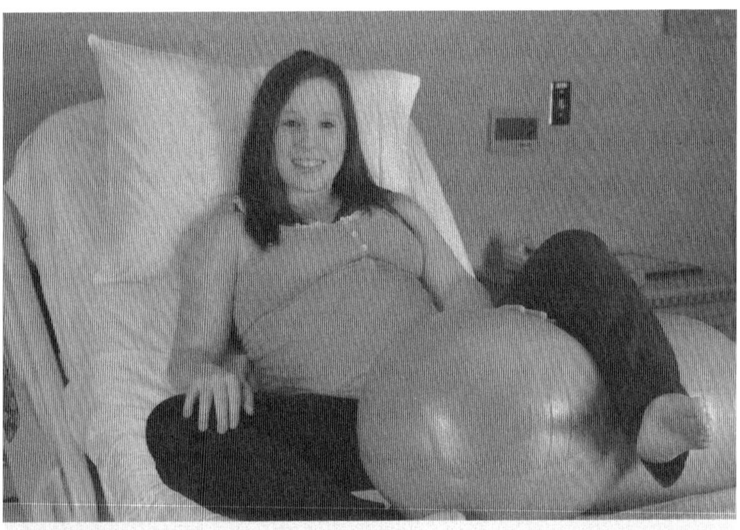

External rotation, knees out. 40 cm peanut ball. *Photo © Premier Birth Tools LLC*

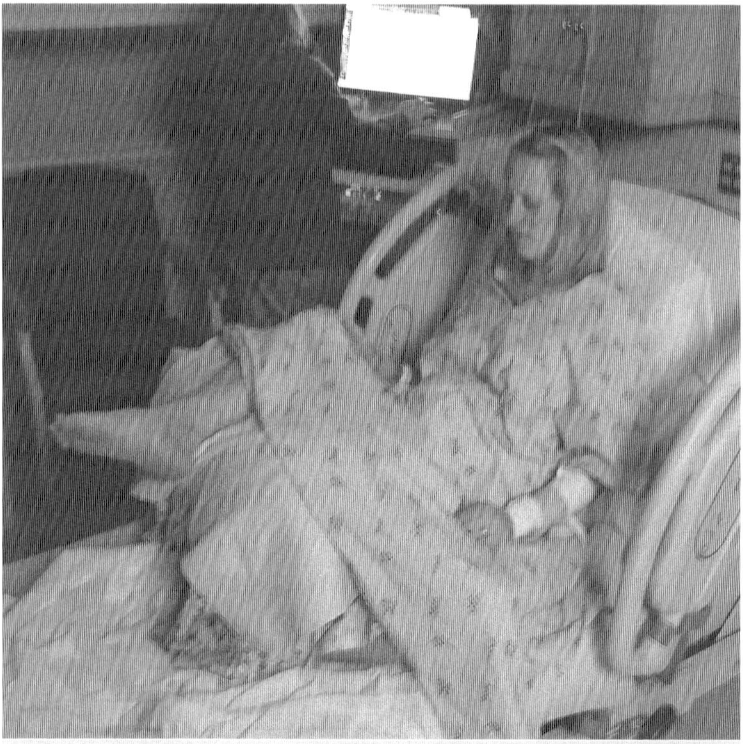

Cover ball. *Photo © Premier Birth Tools LLC*

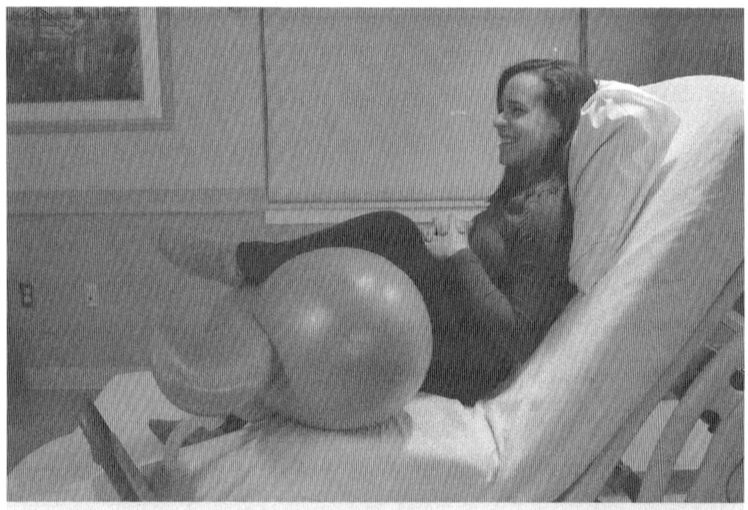

Side view. Use Stirrup to stabilize ball. *Photo courtesy of Amy Bookwalter, CD*

Side Lying on Peanut Ball

In Side-Lying Position, the peanut ball is placed between the client's legs while lying on their side. The peanut ball should be angled so the upper leg is around the indention, or narrow part, and aligned with both knee and ankle resting on the ball.

- Place peanut ball between client's legs, while lying on side, with the top leg over the indention
- Make sure client is turned all the way on their side. Their back should not be flat on the bed.

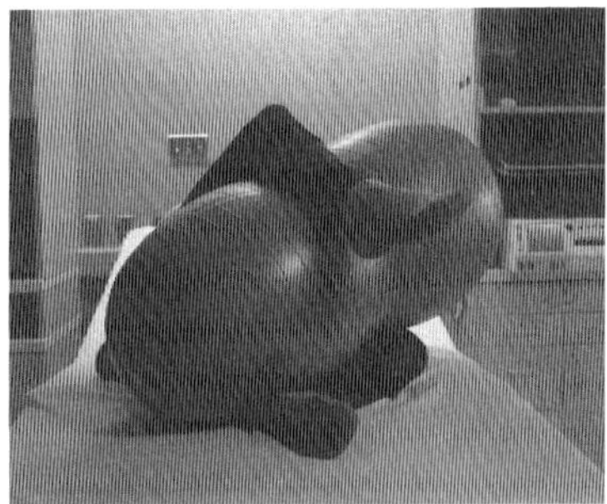

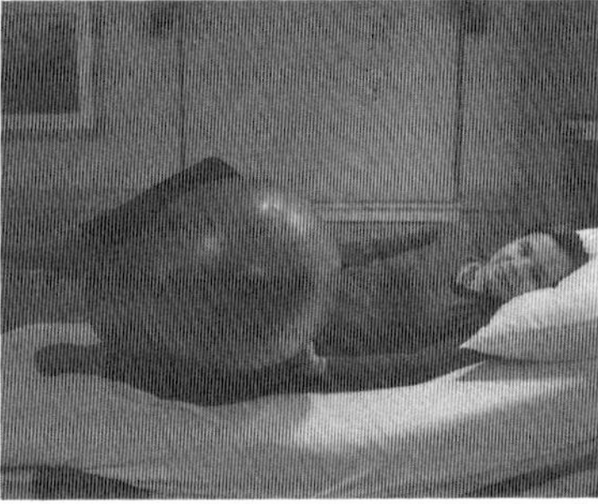

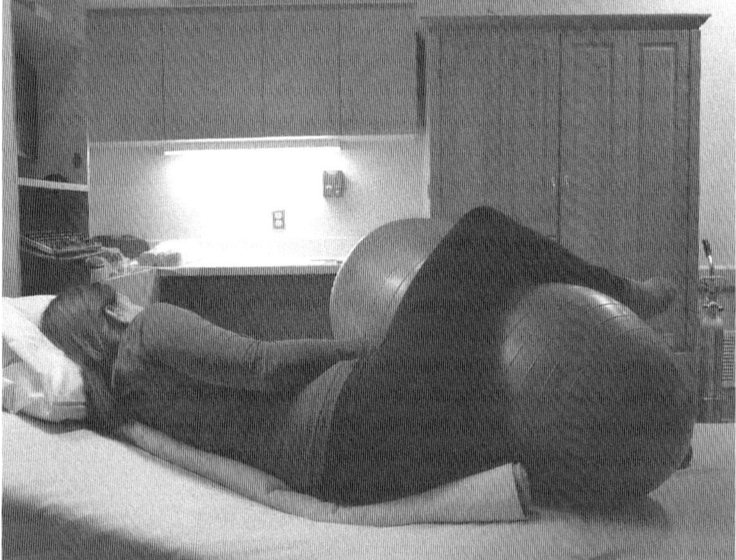

External rotation of femur or thigh bone knees out.

Photos courtesy of Amy Bookwalter, CD

Caution: *Size client correctly.* I see nurses laying clients on their side and calling it a Side-Lying Position, as they use whatever size peanut ball they can find. The client's pelvis is twisted in a rotation that is not purposeful. It's important to size each client for the correct size of peanut ball.

Here is an exception for this particular client's needs: On this client a 50 cm peanut ball is used. This works for external rotation. It would be too big for neutral or internal rotation. A different size ball is used on the same client for different needs and positions. Determine your client's individual needs.

Side-Lying Squat

In Side-Lying Squat Position, femur or thigh bone (top leg) is internally rotated with a towel under top ankle. The bottom leg is internally rotated or neutral, like client is squatting on the peanut ball.

- Place peanut ball between client's legs, while lying on side, with the top leg over the indention
- Make sure client is turned all the way on their side. Their back should not be flat on the bed
- Femur or thigh bone of the the top leg is internally rotated with a towel under the top ankle

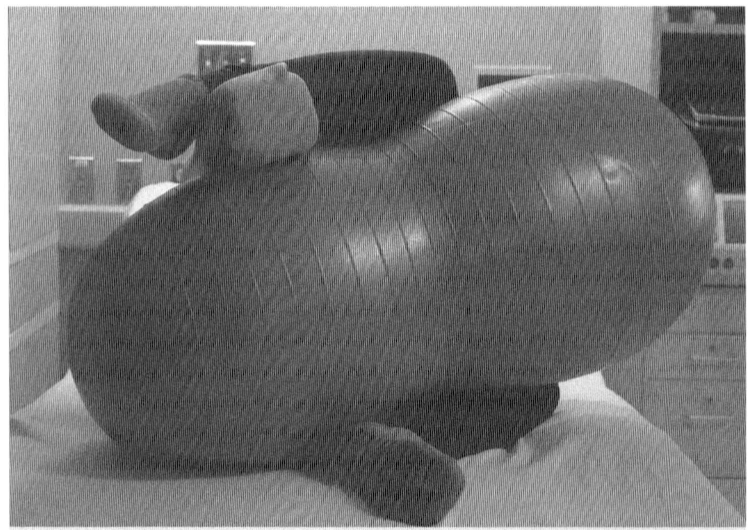

Photo courtesy of Amy Bookwalter, CD

Straddling the Bed Leaning on the Peanut Ball

This position allows the client to rest, straddling the bed. It allows for inlet position; knees are pointed outward and heels towards the ball.

- Client straddles bed
- Choose correct size of ball for client to lean forward and rest

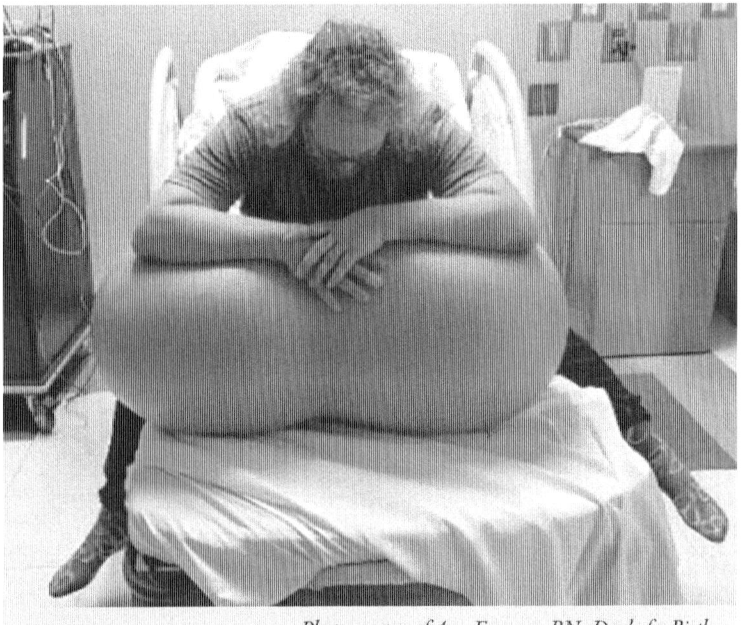

Photo courtesy of Amy Emerson, RN, Doula for Birth

Straddling the Peanut Ball

This position allows the client to rest, straddling the peanut ball. It also allows movement in two planes—a forward to backward movement (primary movement) and an up and down (secondary movement). The saddle shape in the center of the ball cradles and supports the client laterally, giving them more stability. The more supported they feel, the more they will relax. It encourages a squatting position with support. Use only the 70 cm peanut ball in this position, as the other sizes are too small. For inlet position, make sure knees are pointed outward and heels are towards the ball.

- Place client straddling peanut ball
- Only use 70 cm peanut ball to sit on; use a hospital grade peanut ball
- Use another peanut ball to rest head on

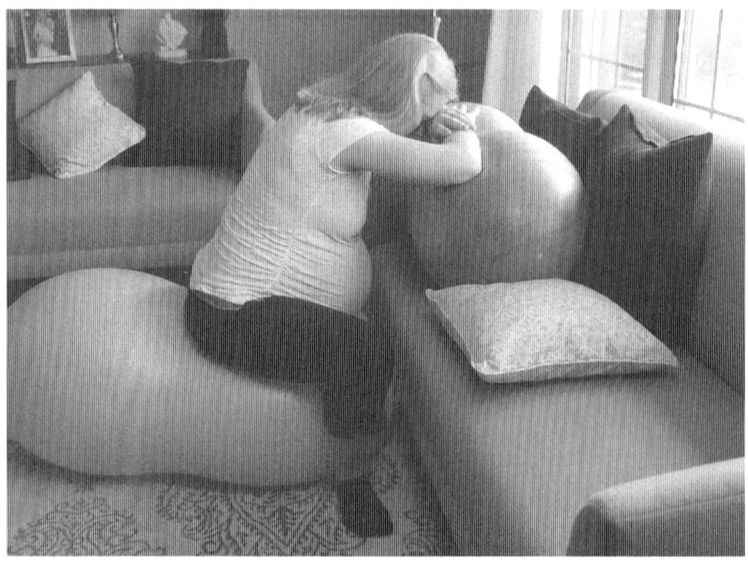

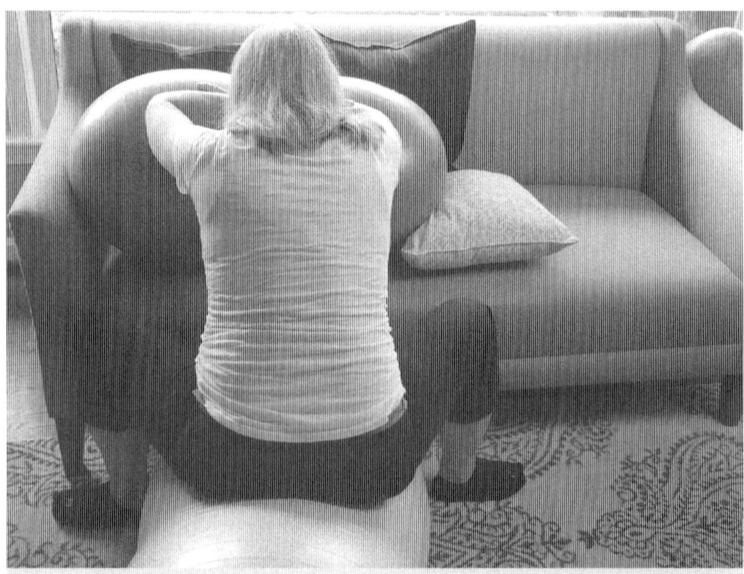

At home, forward resting external rotation of femur bones opens the *top* of the pelvis. *Photos courtesy of Amy Bookwalter, CD*

Straddling with Support

This position allows the client to rest, straddling the peanut ball, with support. The client's partner or doula can sit behind the peanut ball for support. It encourages a squatting position with support. Use only the 70 cm peanut ball in this position, as the other sizes are too small. For inlet position, make sure knees are pointed outward and heels are towards the ball.

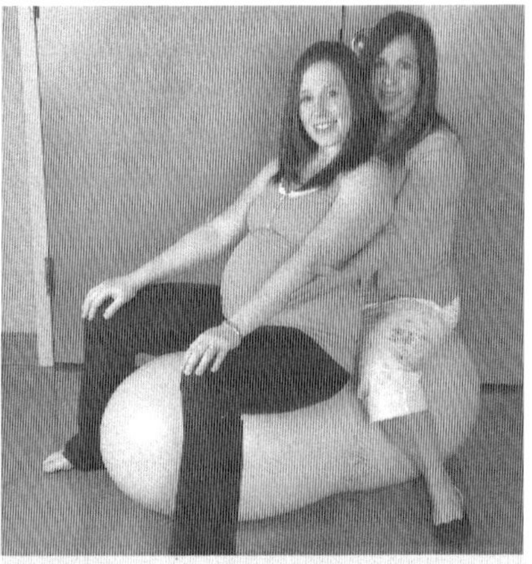

Photo © Premier Birth Tools LLC

- Place client straddling peanut ball
- Only use 70 cm peanut ball to sit on; use a hospital grade peanut ball
- Use with two people for more support

Sitting with Legs on Peanut Ball

Sitting with legs on peanut ball, with external rotation of femur, opens the inlet. This is a wonderful postion to also use with an epidural.

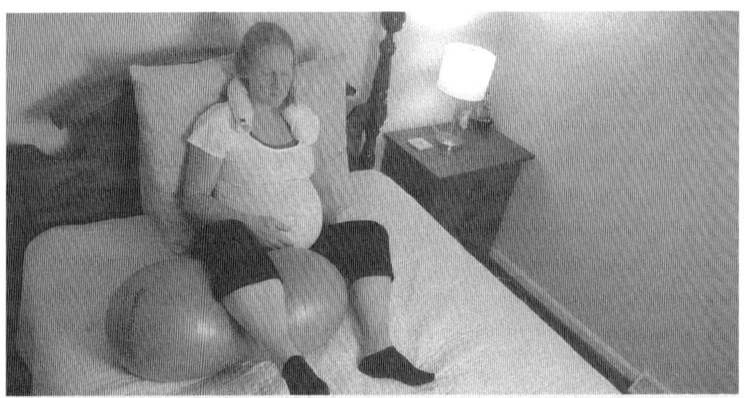

Inlet is external rotation of femur or thigh bone.

Photo courtesy of Amy Bookwalter, CD

OTHER INLET POSITIONS TO USE

There are many more positions. Remember, the clients' knees are pointed outward, heels together, toes out, sitting with knees apart, feet together.

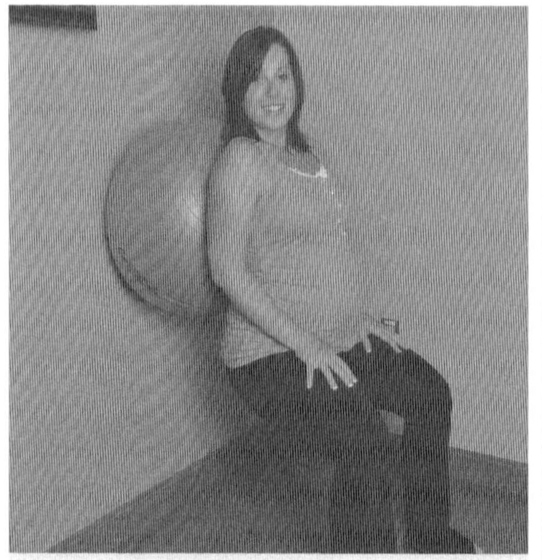

Leaning against the wall.

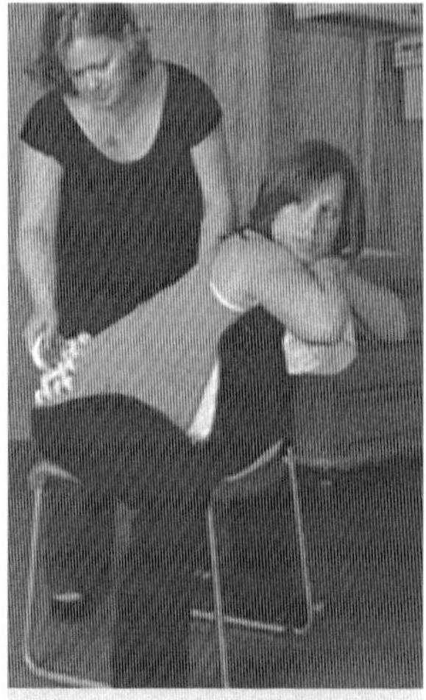

Sitting backwards in a chair.

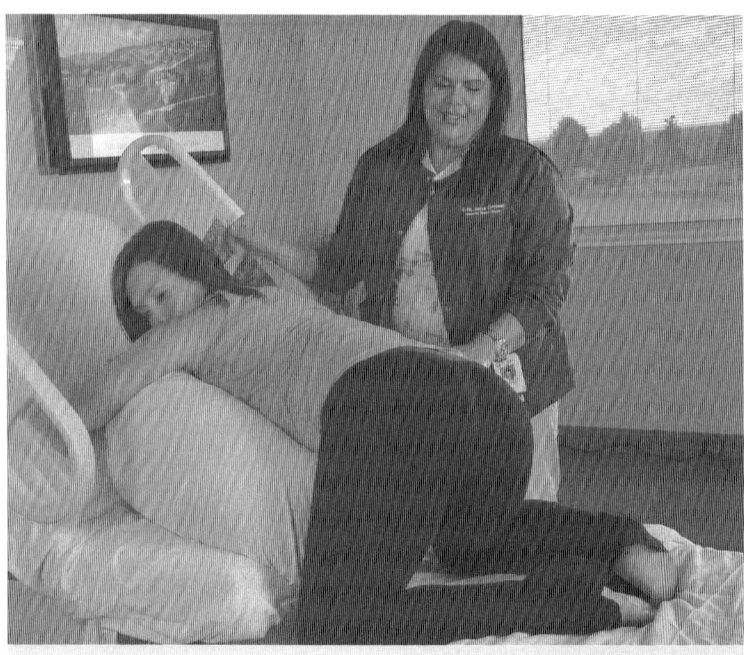

Hands and knees on a bean bag. *Photos © Premier Birth Tools LLC*

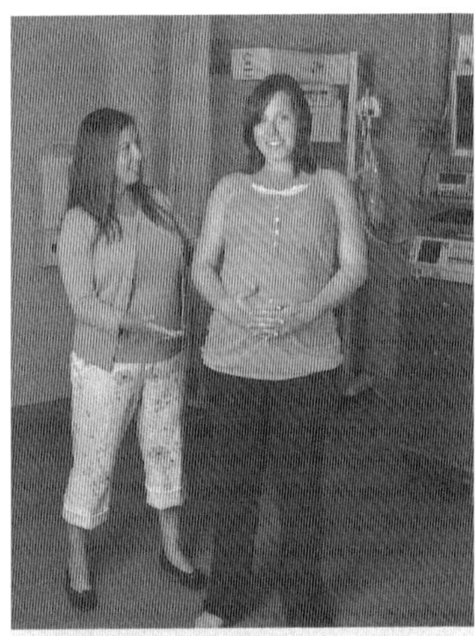

Abdominal lift and tuck.

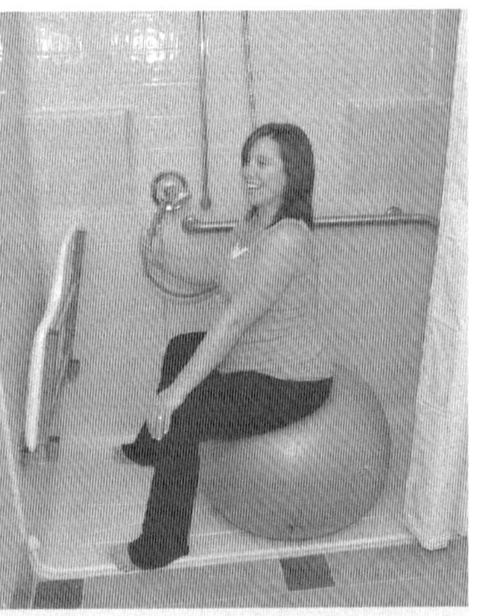

Sitting on ball in shower.

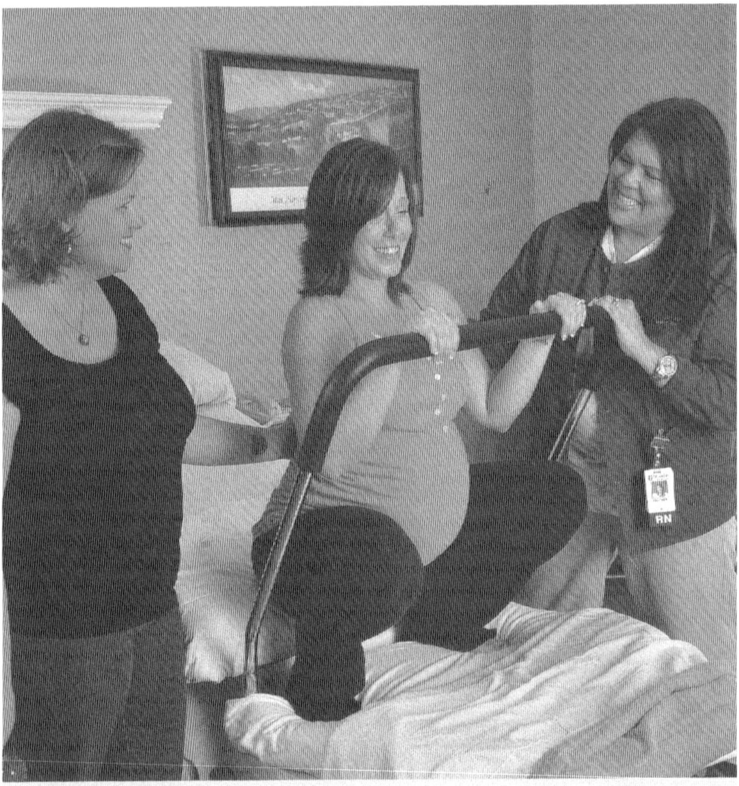

Squat bar. *Photos © Premier Birth Tools LLC*

Inlet—Baby In

External rotation of femur thigh bones = Inlet = Get baby in

External opens **top of pelvis**

Knees pointing outward= Knees Out

Heels together in and toes pointing out in opposite directions

Knees pointing outward—Opens inlet top of pelvis

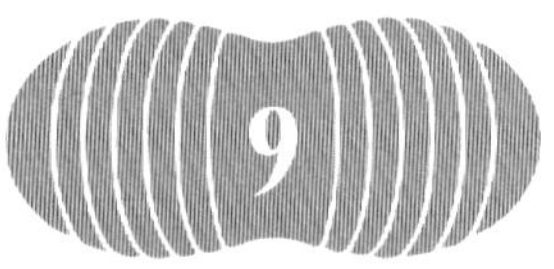

POSITIONS FOR MIDPELVIS

"I have seen the peanut ball work multiple times. I use it on every patient after an epidural and also on some unblocked patients!"

—Brandi Patrick, nurse and Peanut Ball Trainer, Missouri

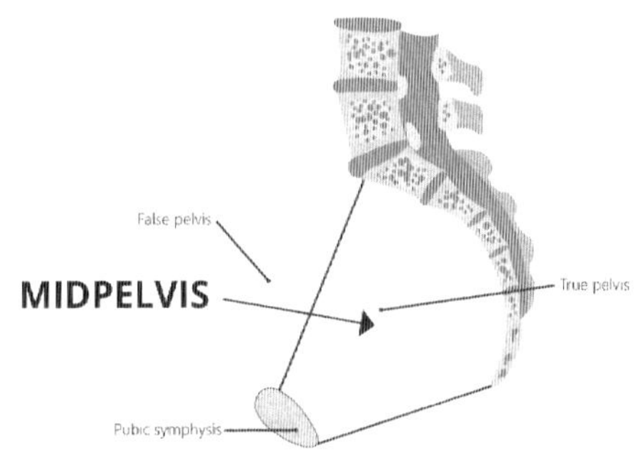

MIDPELVIS MIDDLE OF PELVIS

Neutral, Internal, and External rotation make room for baby to TURN in the pelvis

Midpelvis - Baby Turn
Neutral or internal rotation of femur thighbones =Midpelvis = Get baby to turn
Neutral opens Middle of pelvis
Knees pointing Straight, Heels Straight and Toes Straight
Knees Pointing Straight—Opens Midpelvis—Middle of pelvis

POSITIONS FOR MIDPELVIS

The midpelvis opens in the middle, or narrowest part, of the pelvis. The baby turns on the pelvic floor and enters the narrow part of the pelvis, engaging -1, 0, +1 station. The widest part of the pelvis is located at a diagonal diameter. It opens front to back midpelvis. Movement includes: sideways, diagonal, and uneven hip, including lunges and peanut ball movements. Create a rotation in the pelvis that opens diagonally. Sideways movements open pelvis floor side to side to allow rotation and descent. Nikki Zerfas states, "I want to point out that widening the space between the ischial spines is what helps to open this level of the pelvis, which is why using asymmetric positions is so helpful in the midpelvis."

Knee Position: *When using midpelvis positions, knees are pointing straight, toes are neutral or parallel, and femur or thigh bone is neutral.* An easy way to remember, thanks to Amy Bookwalter, CD, is like parallel windshield wipers. When the client is sitting on the peanut ball, or standing with their feet and knees parallel to each other, rotate back and forth like a windshield-wiper motion.

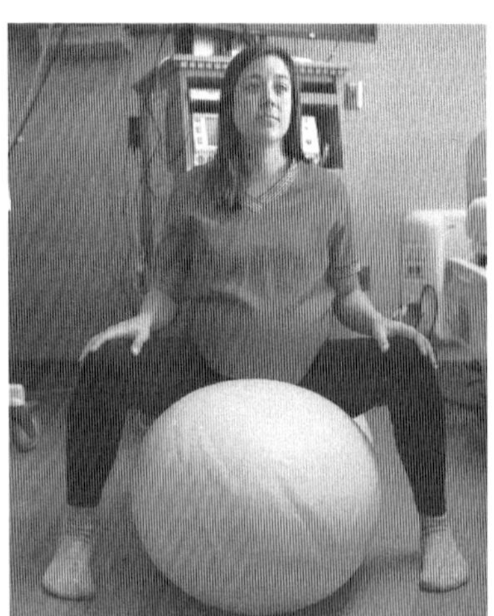

Knees Pointing Straight—Midpelvis.
Photo © Premier Birth Tools LLC

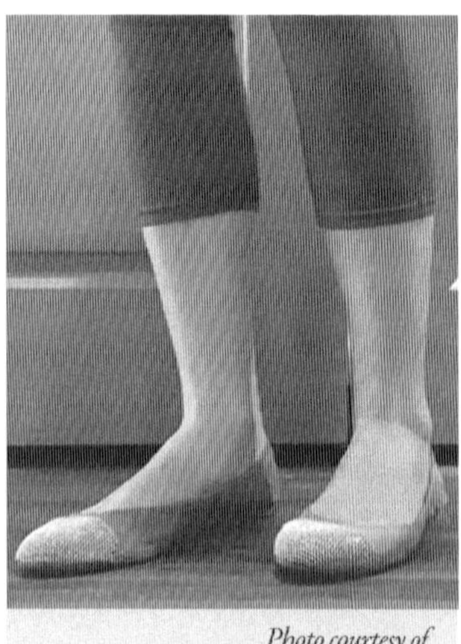

Photo courtesy of Megan E. Honaker, RN, DNP

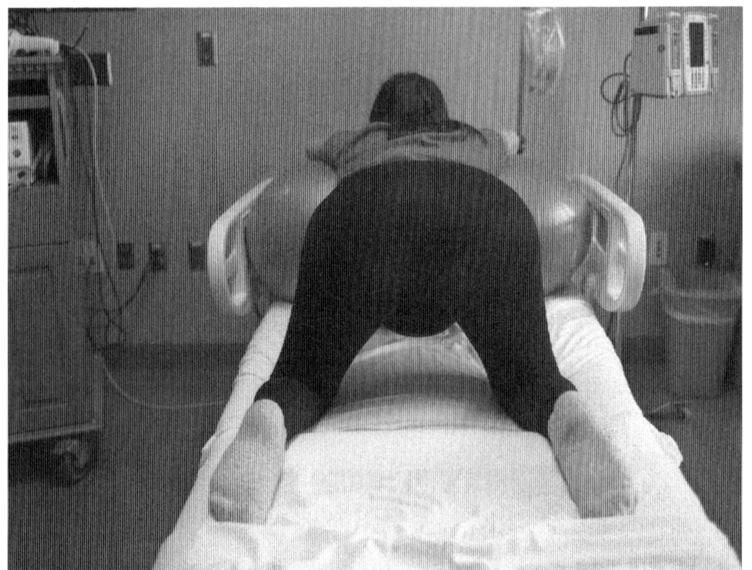

When baby is in the midpelvis, knees pointing forward in a wide neutral position.

Photo © Premier Birth Tools LLC

Hands and Knees

Resting on the peanut ball provides comfort, and also makes sure the client is hanging the baby so it can turn to the optimal position—especially if occiput posterior or asynclitic. Leaning Forward will provide some gravity advantage and align the fetus with the pelvis. This position will aid in opening the *midpelvis* and in reducing an anterior cervical lip. On hands and knees, the rotation of the femur can change from external, to neutral, to internal by rotating the feet. *Follow the knees*. If the knees is pointing *in*, towards the other knee, that makes for internal rotation. If the knee is pointing *out*, away from the other knee, that leg is doing external rotation.

- Place client on hands and knees and lower bottom of the bed
- Have client lean over the peanut ball
- Hands and knees with knees straight for midpelvis
- Allows baby to navigate through the midpelvis
- *If movement is needed, the client should move both knees at same time, rotating from left, to right, and repeat.*

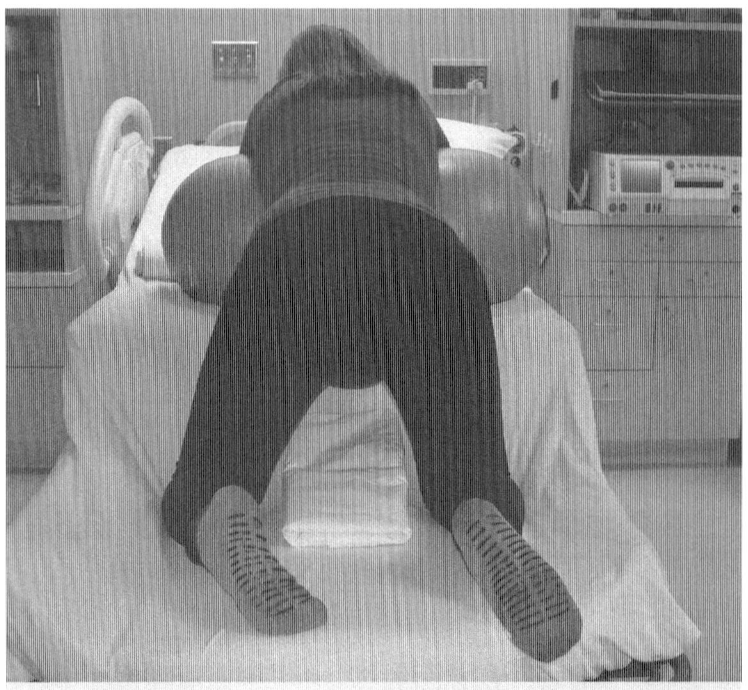

Midpelvis knees parallel and neutral.

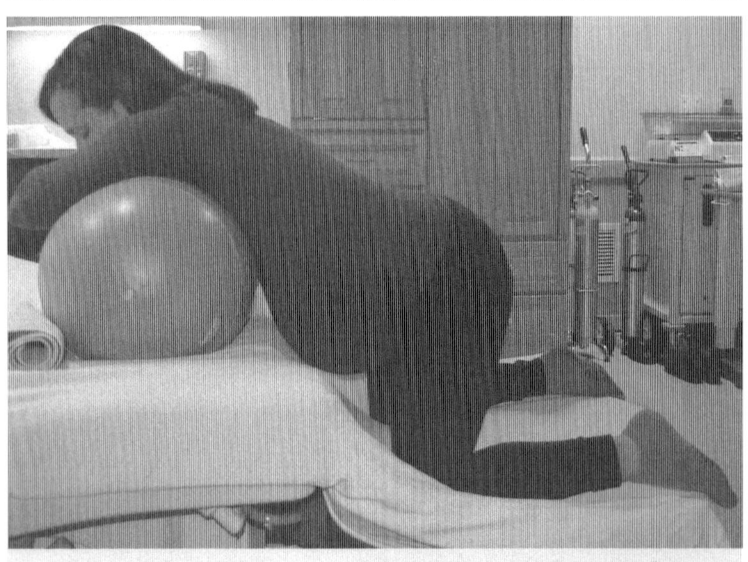

Side view.

Photos courtesy of Amy Bookwalter, CD

Side-Lying Parallel Position

This position assists in opening for fetal rotation of femur or thigh bone, and is all about opening sideways, diagonal, and uneven. The goal is to mimic a side, or diagonal, lunge by rolling towards the belly.

- Place client on their side with peanut ball between their legs
- Point knees straight forward, parallel, and neutral; switch sides frequently

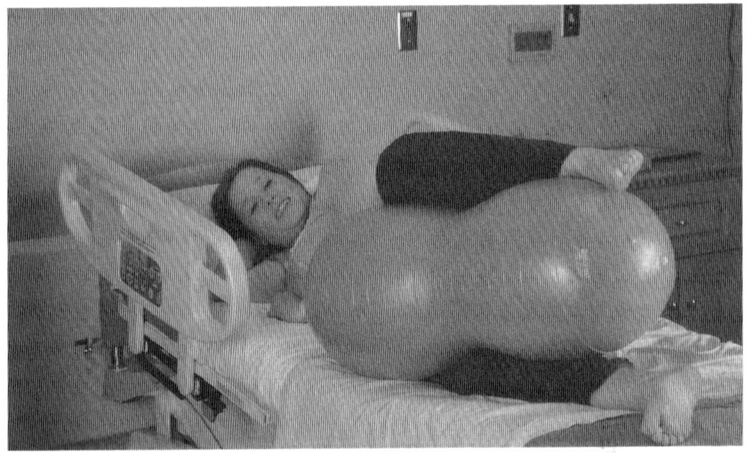

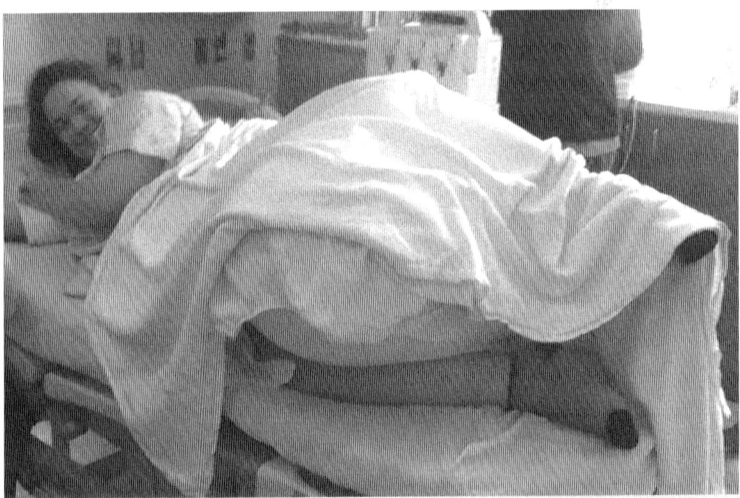

Lying on side with peanut ball between legs.

Photo courtesy of Marlita Camacho

Sitting with Legs on Peanut Ball

Sitting with legs on peanut ball, with internal external rotation of femur, opens the Midpelvis. This is a wonderful postion to also use with an epidural.

- Internal rotation of femur or thigh bone and external rotation of femur or thigh bone happens when adding motion of the knees, rocking or turning back and forth. This becomes the Rocking the Boat Position. *See page 105 for detailed information on this position.*
- Left leg of femur or thigh bone is external rotation
- Right leg of femur or thigh bone is internal rotation
- Feet are placed like windshield wipers

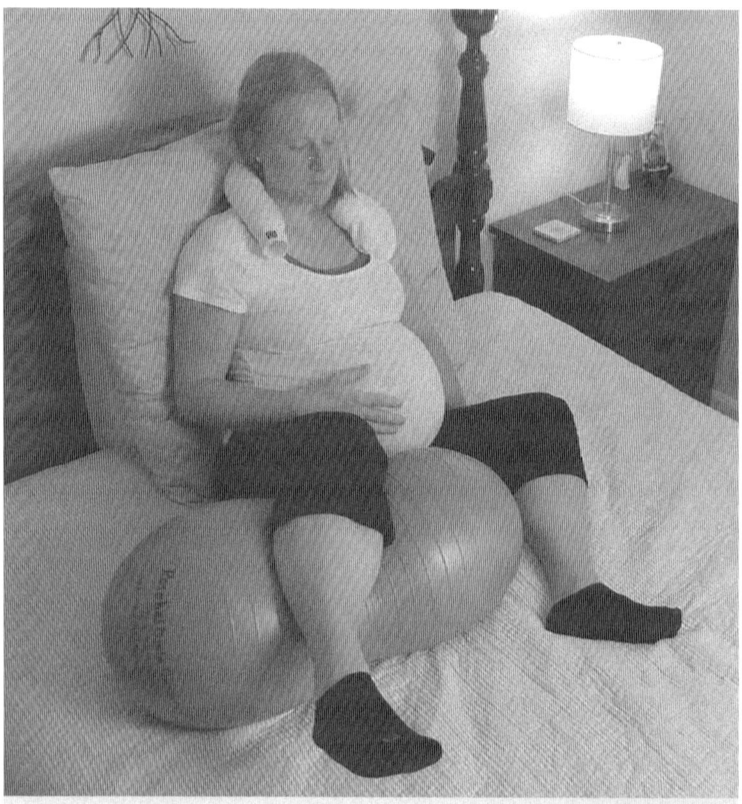

Opens midpelvis Left leg is externally rotated, right leg is internally rotated.

Photo courtesy of Amy Bookwalter, CD

Side-Lying Lunge (Runner's Position)

This position encourages the baby to move up and reposition its head, tuck its chin, and come back down. This position will slightly torque the client's pelvis, close the bottom of the outlet, and will open the inlet to make more or less room in that area of the pelvis. This position has several different names: Texas Roll, Runners, Exaggerated Sims, Semi-Prone, and more.

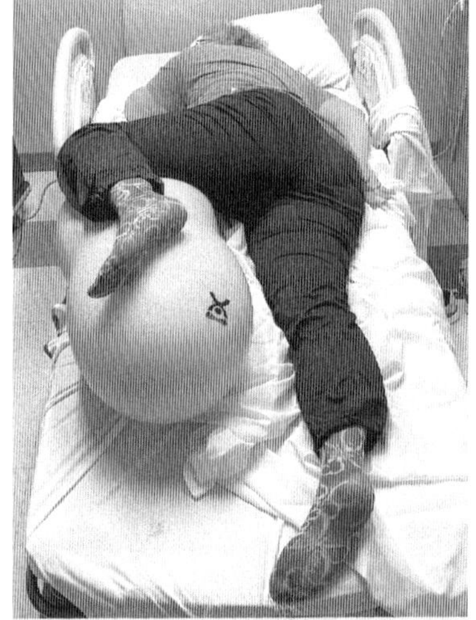

Runner's Position.

- This position is the same as lunging
- The bottom leg is straight. The other leg is bent 90 degrees with the foot over and in front of peanut ball, while lying on side
- The upper body needs to rotate so the chest is facing down on the bed, as if trying to sleep on stomach
- Turn client to the side more toward her stomach, as tolerated, with upper leg bent inside towards the chest
- Upper front arm is bent at the elbow, positioned comfortably in front of the body
- Back arm is straight behind client, close to the buttocks
- Laying with the baby's back towards the ceiling will help gravity to turn the baby

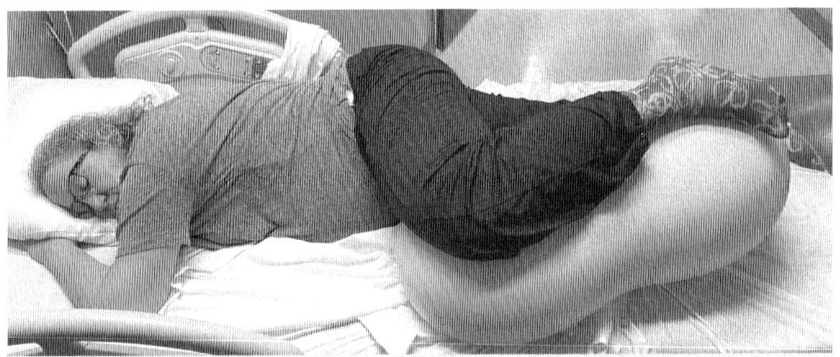

Photos courtesy of Amy Emerson, RN, Doula For Birth

Forward Leaning

Lower the bottom of the bed, then have the client lean over the peanut ball on their hands and knees. Resting on the peanut ball provides comfort and also makes sure the client is hanging the baby so it can turn to the optimal position—especially if occiput posterior or asynclitic. Leaning Forward will provide some gravity advantage and align the baby with the pelvis. This position will aid in opening the midpelvis. Ensure the knees are pointed straight. This position may also help reduce an anterior cervical lip.

- Place client on hands and knees, lying over peanut ball and lower the bottom of the bed
- Have client lean over the peanut ball
- Knees parallel and straight

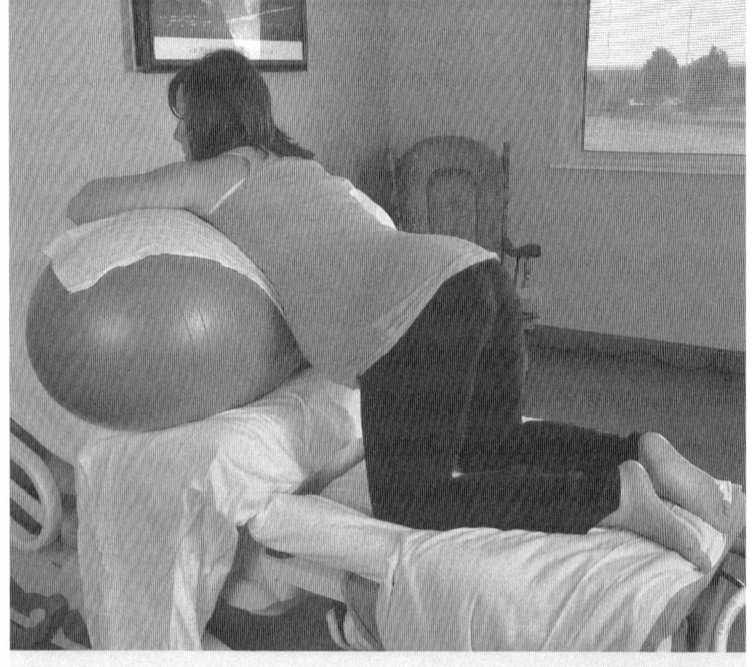

Photo © Premier Birth Tools LLC

Rock the Boat

By Tammy Ryan, SpBT

This position opens and keeps movement in the midpelvis. The rocking helps to rock the ischial spine back and forth, so the baby can rotate past the ischial spine. This is helpful when the client is in the bed with an epidural or wants to rest, because the peanut ball will help maintain movement of the pelvis to help with fetal descent and/or rotation during labor. The goal is to mimic a side or diagonal lunge by rolling towards the belly.

Tammy Ryan, SpBT, states, "The leg should be in a 90-degree angle (femur is on the opposite side of the ischial spine), supporting both knee and ankle with the ball. *By rocking the peanut ball back and forth you keep constant motion in the midpelvis at the ischial spines to help baby rotate through.* It is a great midpelvis solution!"

- Client is lateral and the peanut ball is parallel to the bottom leg. The top leg rests on a peanut ball with the knee bent at a 90 degree angle. Gently roll the femur or thigh bone on the peanut ball, rocking side to side as the ball would naturally roll. The bottom leg can also be straight
- Use this position for 30 minutes on each side of the peanut ball in front of stomach, with doula or partner rocking the peanut ball
- The peanut ball can create a lot of tension on the pubic symphysis while rotating the femurs and pelvis out of alignment. Be sure to use the proper size of peanut ball to reduce the possibility of tension. Be careful when using the rocking motion—always use a gentle rocking movement
- Diagonal movement can be created by rolling the lower leg with the peanut ball as a single unit
- Hold both the ankle and knee, and move the entire lower leg together on the peanut ball. This will help facilitate the diagonal movement a client would have if she was standing and lunging, or swaying

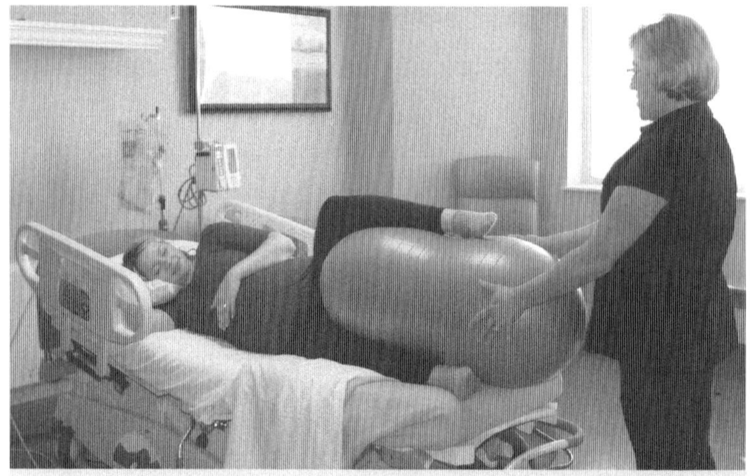

Rock the Boat: Top leg at 90 degrees.

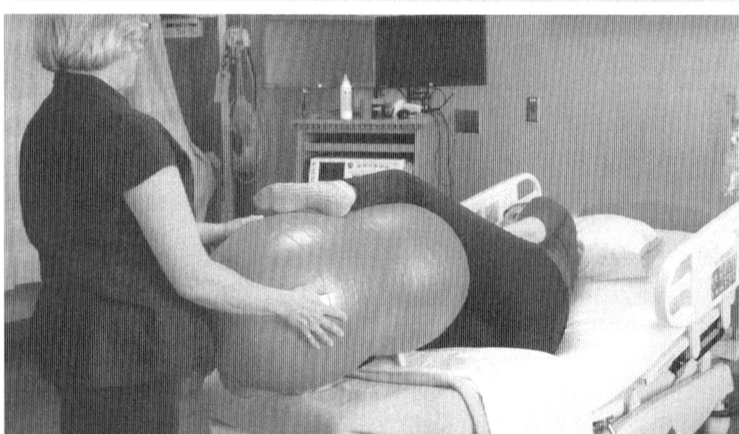

Rocking peanut ball side to side.

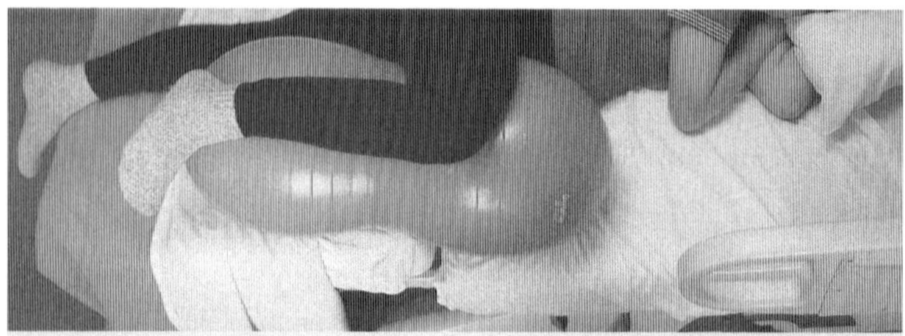

Keep leg at a 90-degree angle when rocking the boat.

Photos © Premier Birth Tools LLC

Fire Hydrant

By Cheri Grant, RN, Premier Birth Tools

On hands and knees, place one leg on top of peanut ball with other leg kneeling. This opens half of the pelvis, mid and outlet. Then place the peanut ball on the lower portion of the bed with the client's leg on the peanut ball in a Fire Hydrant Position or Kneeling Lunge. This position may aid in reducing an anterior cervical lip. It also widens the midpelvis to make room for the baby to rotate—for instance, if in an occiput transverse position. The Fire Hydrant position is challenging for the client to keep stable. Be sure to use bed railings, people positioned beside her, towels, stirrups, or bean bag chairs to support her position.

- Place the client on hands and knees and lower the bottom of the bed
- You can use a bean bag under the client's belly to support the client for comfort—especially one with an epidural. Make sure the client is hanging the baby so it can turn to the optimal position. *See page 51*
- Place the client's leg on the peanut ball in a Fire Hydrant Position.
- Use a stirrup to hold the ball in place, use bed rails, and have someone stand by for support
- I use the name "Fire Hydrant "(Grant, Chart 2013), and Gail Tully, CPM, Spinning Babies® named it the Kneeling Lunge (Tully, Drawing 2014). *See Fun Fact below*
- Same as Kneeling Lunge on following pages

Fun Fact

After I spoke at the 2014 LAMAZE/DONA conference on peanut balls. Gail Tully CPM Spinning Babies® and I were brainstorming additional new peanut ball positions. When Gail drew this picture, she named it the Kneeling Lunge. I had just presented and published it in an article and called it the Fire Hydrant Position (Clutter, Grant 2014 12-15). They are the same position just different names.

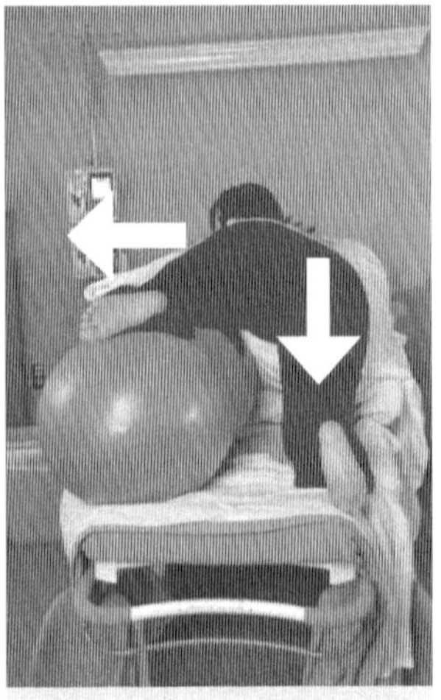

Fire Hydrant.
Photo © Premier Birth Tools LLC

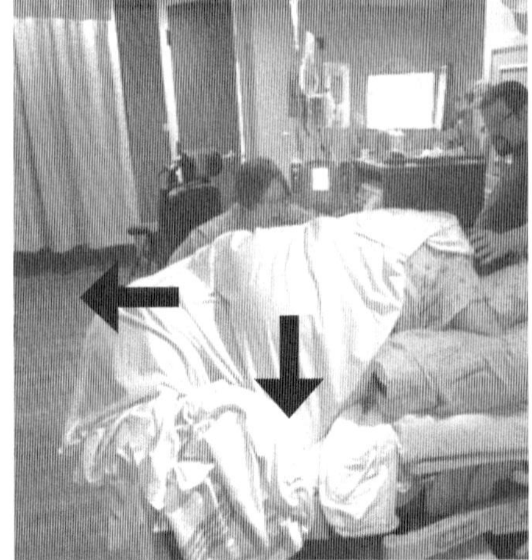

Client with epidural.
Photo courtesy of Sarah Coffin

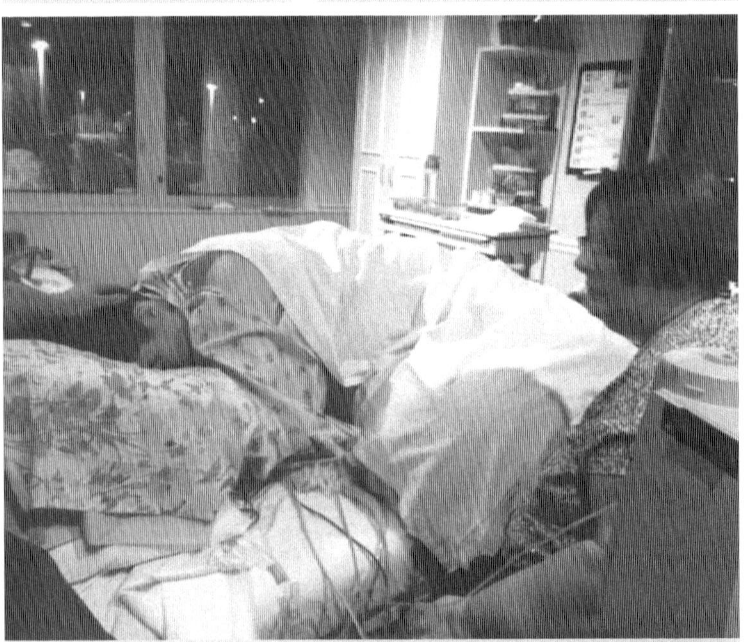

Cheri encourages client with an epidural.
Photo courtesy of Sarah Coffin

Note: *Some nurses call a leg in the stirrup or overbed table Fire Hydrant. This is* **not** *the same effect when used with a peanut ball.*

Kneeling Lunge (AKA Fire Hydrant)

By Gail Tully, CPM, Spinning Babies®

This position provides some gravity advantage and aligns the baby with the pelvis, aiding in internal and external rotation of femur or thigh bone through opening half of the midpevis. It may also help reduce an anterior cervical lip.

- Place the client on hands and knees and lower the bottom of the bed
- Place the peanut ball on the lower portion of the bed with the client's leg on the peanut ball in a fire hydrant pose
- Same as Fire Hydrant
- I use the name "Fire Hydrant" (Grant, 2013) and Gail Tully, CPM, Spinning Babies®, named it the Kneeling Lunge (Tully Drawing, 2014)

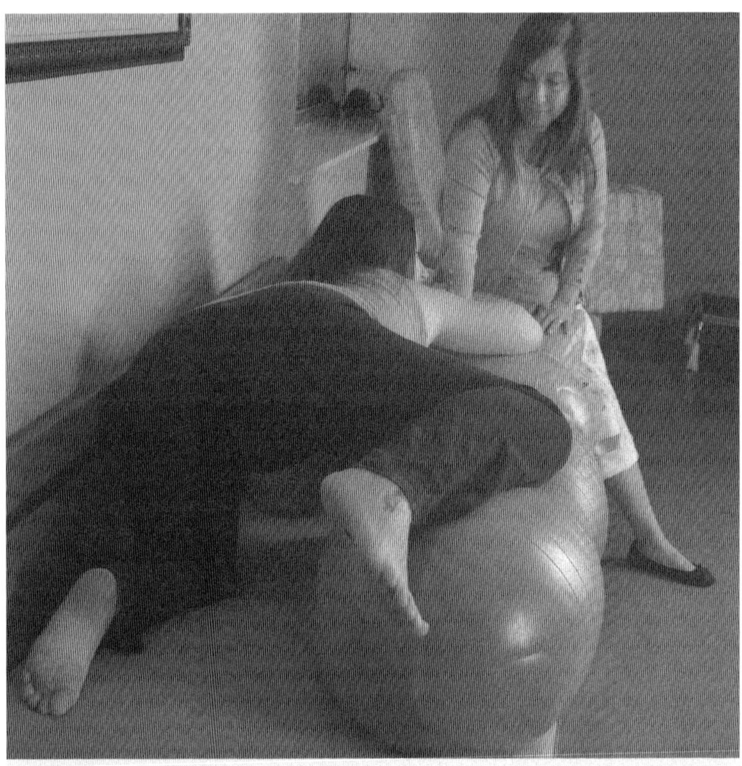

Photo © Premier Birth Tools LLC

Double Peanut Ball

By Sarah Lavonne, RN, Bundle Birth

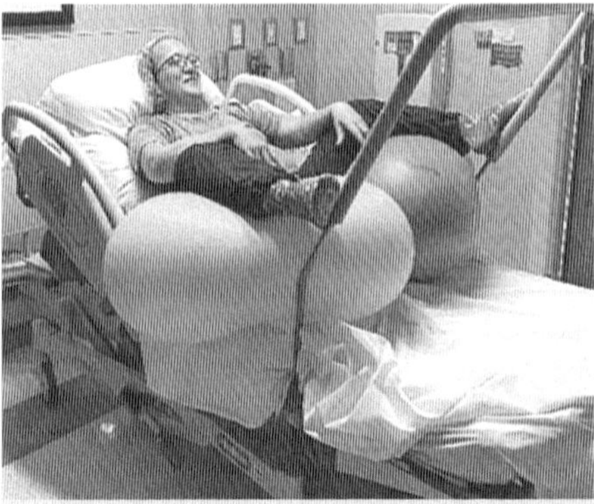
Photo courtesy of Amy Emerson, Doula for Birth

This position is for mid-pelvis. Resting with feet on squat bar and peanut balls under legs.

- Place squat bar on bed
- Rest legs on peanut ball with feet resting on squat bar

Tuck Position

By Cheri Grant, RN, Premier Birth Tools

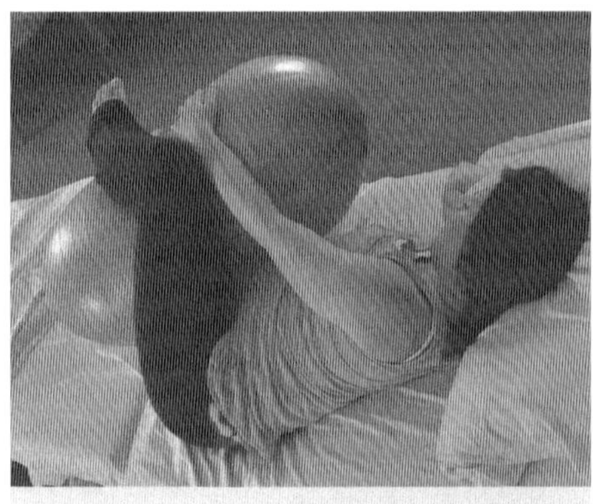
Photo © Premier Birth Tools LLC

The Tuck Position is one of the most important and efficient positions. It can help to rotate a posterior positioned baby to a more optimal fetal position, and allows the baby to descend when in the midpelvis. Tuck is also a wonderful pushing position, which is discussed later in the book.

- Place the peanut ball, as high as possible, between the client's legs
- Top leg over the indention
- The leg under the ball should be as close to the client's chest as possible
- Bring the peanut ball in close to the client as she is hugging it
- To assist with positioning, the bedrail can be used to hold the ball in place
- Blanket can be put behind the ball and placed behind client's back

OTHER MIDPELVIS POSITIONS

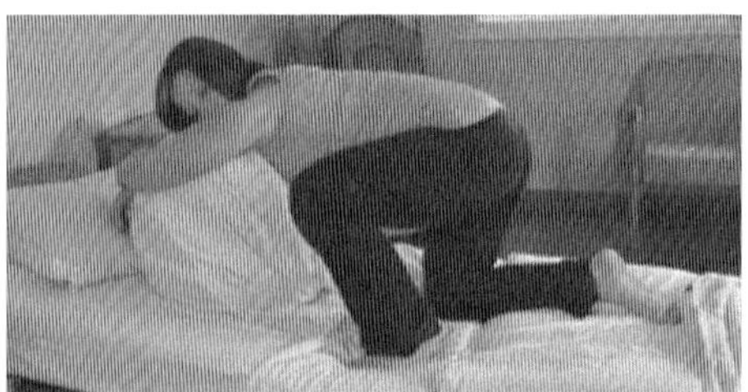

Asymmetrical Lunge Knees Forward

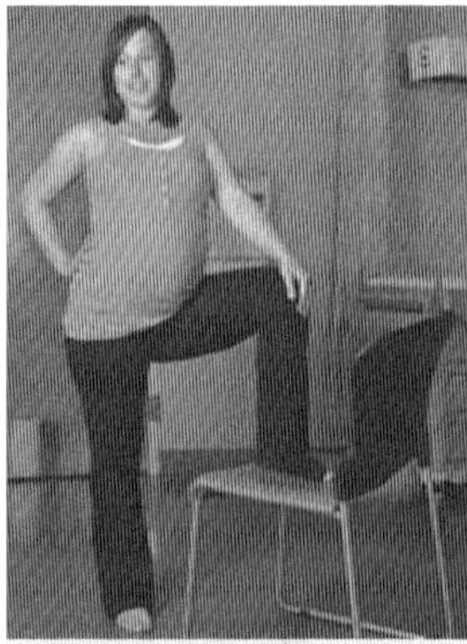

Lunge

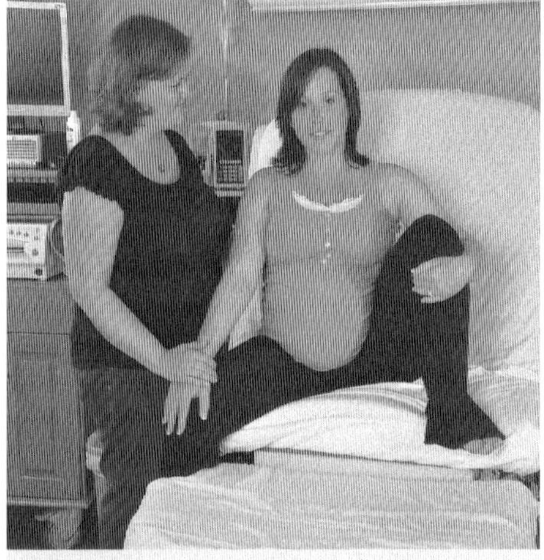

Asymetrical Sitting

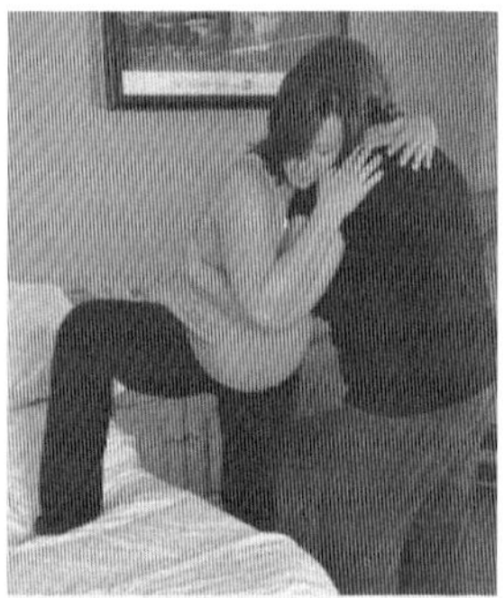

Asymmetrical Standing

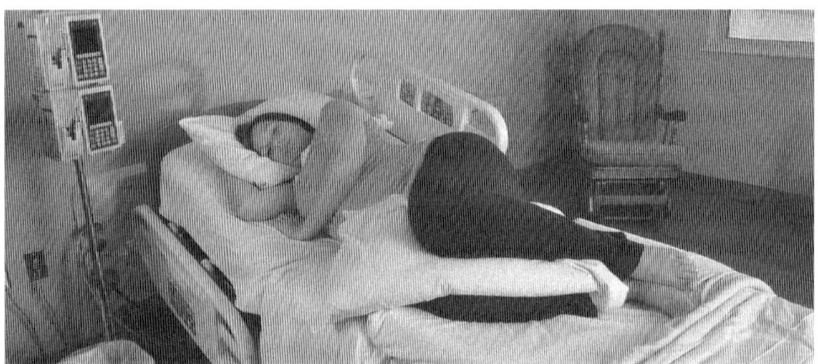

Side-Lying, knees parallel or neutral. *Photos © Premier Birth Tools LLC*

See set of 14 charts for addtional positions at Premier Birth Tools store: premierbirthtools.com.

Midpelvis—Baby Turn

Both internal and external rotation of femur or thigh bone makes room for baby to TURN in pelvis with back and forth motion =

Midpelvis = Get baby to turn

Neutral opens middle of pelvis

Knees pointing straight, heels straight, and toes pointing straight

Knees pointing straight—Opens midpelvis—Middle of pelvis

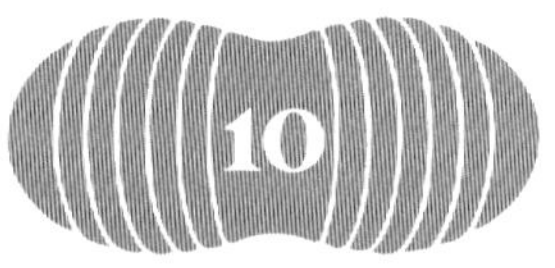

POSITIONS TO OPEN THE OUTLET

"Just wanted to say thanks for the awesome, ever-magical peanut ball! They truly have changed the way I take care of my laboring mamas! Love, love, love the peanut balls!"

—April Montgomery, nurse, Alabama

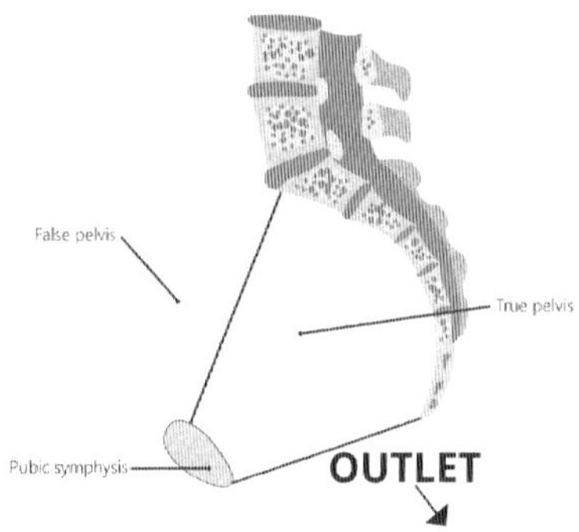

OUTLET BOTTOM OF PELVIS

Internal rotation makes room for baby to come OUT of the pelvis

Outlet—Baby out
Internal rotation of femur thigh bone = Outlet = Get baby out
Internal opens BOTTOM of pelvis
Knees together pointing inward = Knee to knee
Knees in, heels out, and toes turned in pointing together
Knees pointing in—Opens outlet—BOTTOM of pelvis

POSITIONS TO OPEN THE OUTLET

The outlet opens at the bottom of the pelvis by internally rotating the femur or thigh bone. Here, the baby is low in the pelvis and the client is ready to push +2, +3 station or lower—you can see the baby. The most space in the pelvis is from front to back and can be increased with movement of the sacrum and coccyx (tailbone). Open the outlet from side to side, by rotating the femur or thigh bone in an internal rotation, causing the ischial tuberosities (sitz bones) to move farther apart. Knees in, ankles out."

Knee Position: *When using positions to open the outlet, it is important that the client is knee to knee, pointing inward.* Internal rotation of femur or thigh bone causes an opening of the outlet. Amy Bookwalter, CD, has another fun way to remember knee positioning when working to open the outlet: "'Ruby Red Slippers Dorothy Kick' toes together and heels out before the heel click. The motion of pressing the heels outwardly hastens the baby out of the outlet."

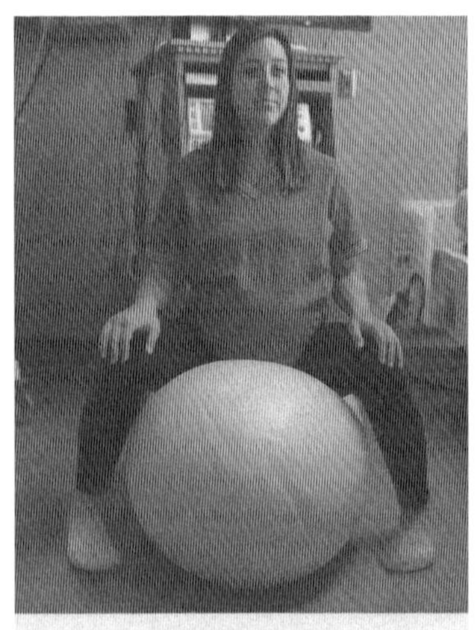

Knees together, outlet.
Photo © Premier Birth Tools LLC

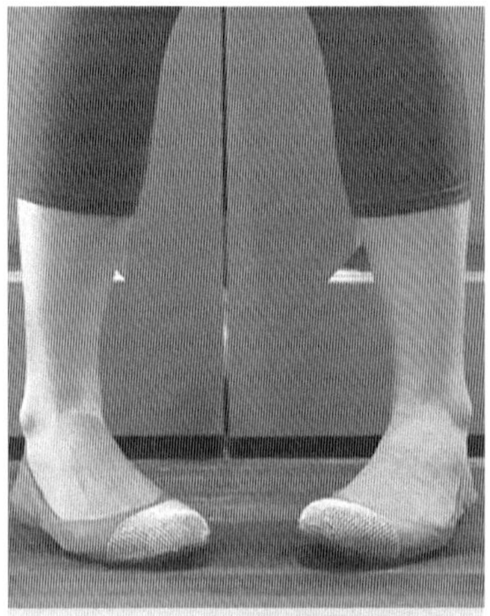

Photo courtesy of Megan E. Honaker, RN, DNP

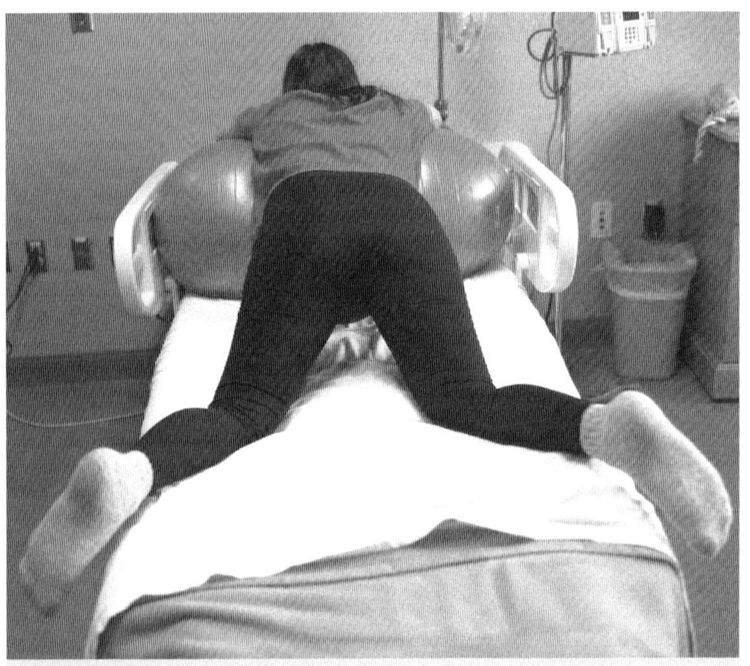

Outlet on peanut ball. Knees together, pointing inward. Internal rotation of femur or thigh bone.
Photo © Premier Birth Tools LLC

With the feet wide, there is internal rotation of the femur or thigh bones that helps open the *bottom* of the pelvis. For internal rotation or thigh bone, to get the baby to the outlet of the pelvis, place the knees together, pointing in, with the feet pointing out (the legs should be in an outward "V" position). In this position, to make even more rotation, the client could put their heels out and toes in, while still in *this* position.

For my students who've had epidurals, the peanut ball has helped some of them maintain external rotation for either the last part of transition or for pushing. For those who have not had an epidural, it's also been helpful as another position to use to facilitate fetal descent into and through the pelvic outlet. Linda Middlekauff, childbirth educator, Oregon

Hand and Knees

Resting on the peanut ball provides comfort and also makes sure the client is hanging the baby so it can turn to the optimal position—especially if occiput posterior or asynclitic. Leaning Forward will provide some gravity advantage and aligns the fetus with the pelvis. On hands and knees, *internal rotation* of the femur or thigh bone happens with knees wide *and feet wide apart*. This position will aid in opening the *outlet* and may help reduce an anterior cervical lip. *Internal rotation* is good for pushing, as it opens the bottom of the pelvis. On hands and knees, the rotation of the femur can change from external, to neutral, to internal, by rotating the feet. *Follow the knees*: if the knee is pointing *in*, towards the other knee, that makes for internal rotation. If the knee is pointing *out*, away from the other knee, that leg is doing external rotation.

- Place client on hands and knees and lower bottom of the bed
- Have client lean over the peanut ball
- *Internal rotation of the* femur or thigh bone happens with knees close together
- In Hands and Knees Postion, the knees are pointing toward each other. The knees can be wide and heels apart
- *Internal rotation* is good for pushing, as it opens the bottom of the pelvis.

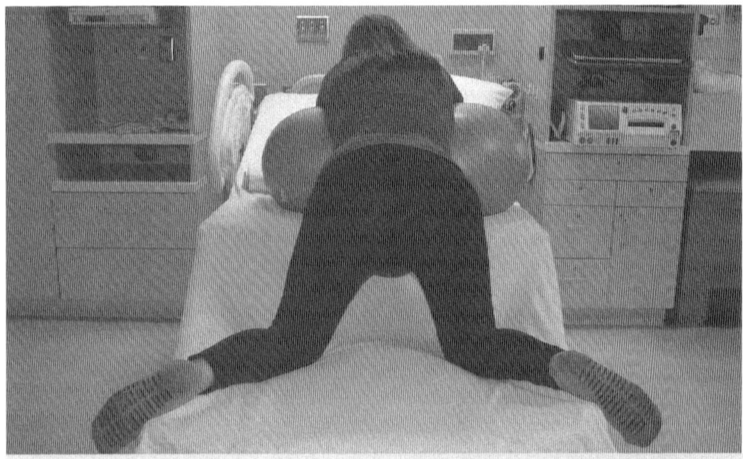

Open outlet: internal rotation of femur or thigh bone with knees wide, feet apart. *Photo courtesy of Amy Bookwalter, CD*

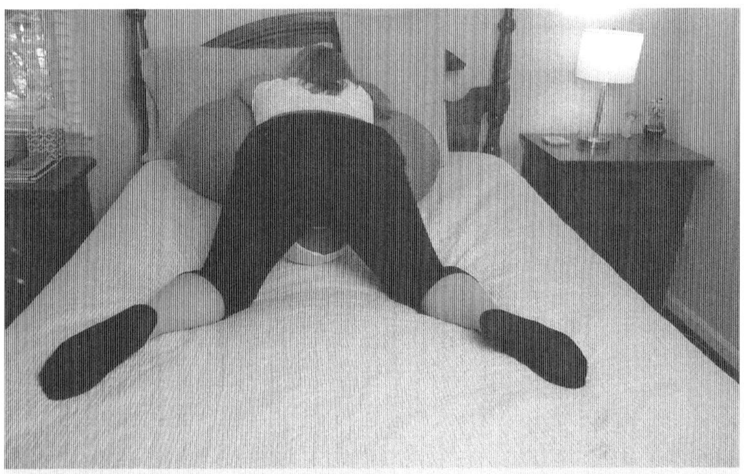

At a home. Open outlet: internal rotation of femur or thigh bone with knees wide, feet apart. *Photo courtesy of Amy Bookwalter, CD*

Straddling Peanut Ball

- Open outlet: internal rotation of femur or thigh bone with knees wide, feet apart
- Knees pointing in opens outlet or bottom of pelvis

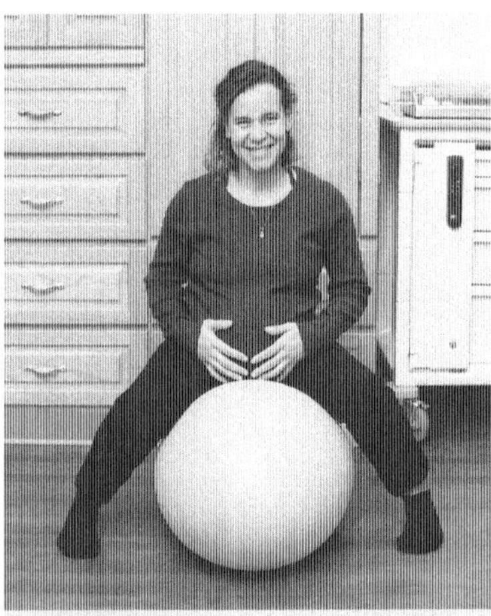

Outlet internal rotation of femur or thigh bone.
Photo courtesy of Amy Bookwalter, CD

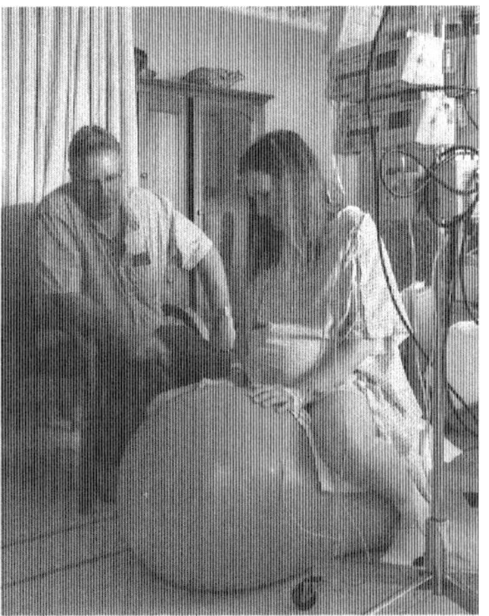

Outlet internal rotation of femur or thigh bone.
Photo courtesy of Samantha Steen, doula and photographer, CLC

Park Bench Sitting

By Gail Tully, CPM, Spinning Babies®

This position is a collaboration between me and Gail Tully, CPM, of Spinning Babies®. Gail created the drawing (Tully Drawing, 2014) and I named the position.

The Park Bench Position gives room for the tailbone anterior pelvic tilt, and moves the sitz bones out, which can flare the tailbone.

- Park Bench gives room for the tailbone anterior pelvic tilt
- Moves the sitz bones out, which can flare the tailbone
- Place feet flat with knees higher than hips and arms lifted, pulling on Rebozo or sheet; ribs are raised
- Lower back, so it is flat, to open the outlet
- Roll back during contraction to arch back
- Tilt tailbone out to open sitz bones
- Roll forward to rest

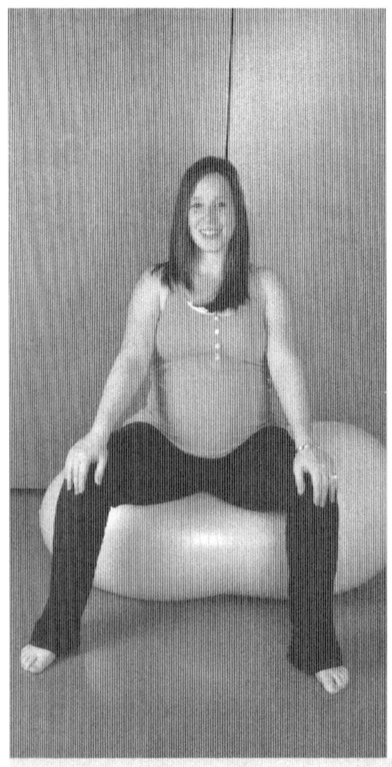

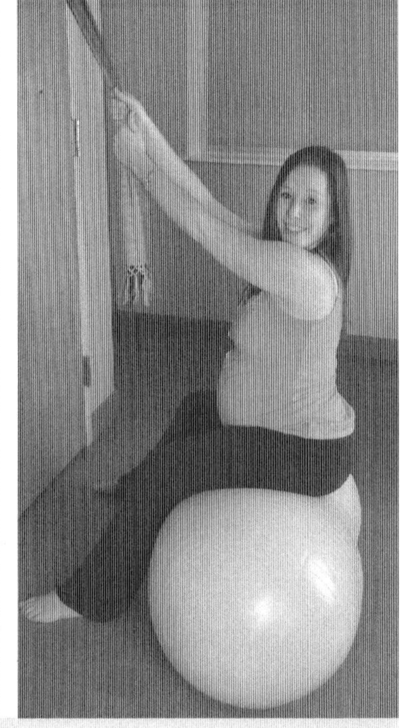

Photo © Premier Birth Tools LLC

Knees Together Heels Out

Popularized in the U.S. by Spinning Babies® Approved Trainers

This position is wonderful to use when the baby is visible or nearly visible. By placing the peanut ball between the ankles, it helps the client ,who may want to rest between pushes or while laboring down. At +2 station, focus on opening the outlet or bottom portion of the pelvis.

Internal rotation of the femur or thigh bone, applied for birth with knees together and heels out, is demonstrated in *Preparing for a Gentle Birth: The Pelvis in Pregnancy* by authors Blandine Callais Germain and Núria Vives Parés (German and Parés, 2012). I highly recommend this book as supplemental reading. Commonly called Knees Together Pushing Position, this position is used during the contraction when baby is low in the pelvis. Turning the toes toward each other rotates the thigh bone to widen the sitz bones. This position was popularized in the U.S. by Spinning Babies® Approved Trainers.

- Knees together with towel between knees, feet apart, and Side -Lying with sitz bones open for baby's head
- Peanut ball is between ankles, internal rotation of the femur or thigh bone, plus knees forward for a neutral spine and sacrum space
- Toes pointed in towards each other and heels out to open lower portion of pelvis

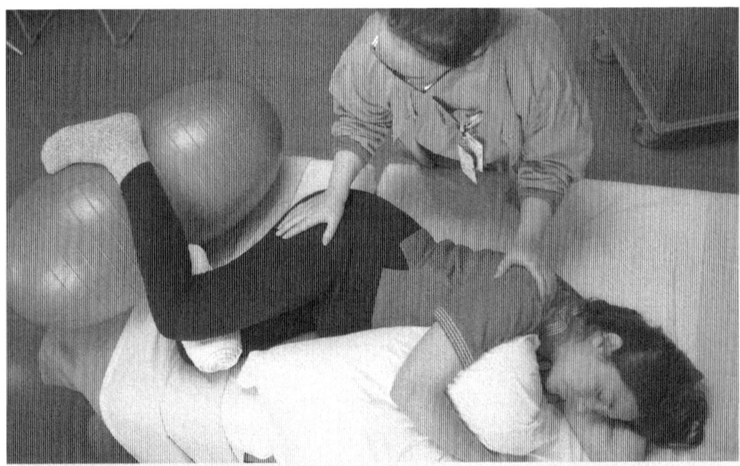

Knees together , Side-Lying with a towel between knees. Sitz bones opens for baby head. *Photo © Premier Birth Tools LLC*

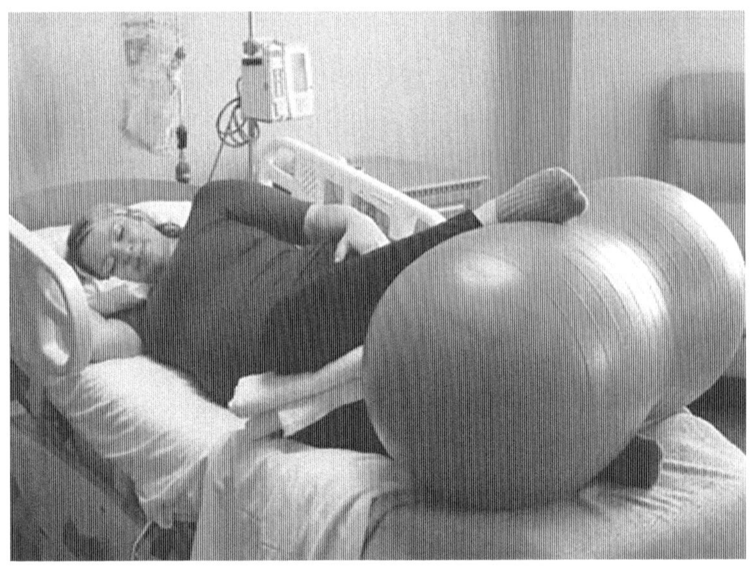

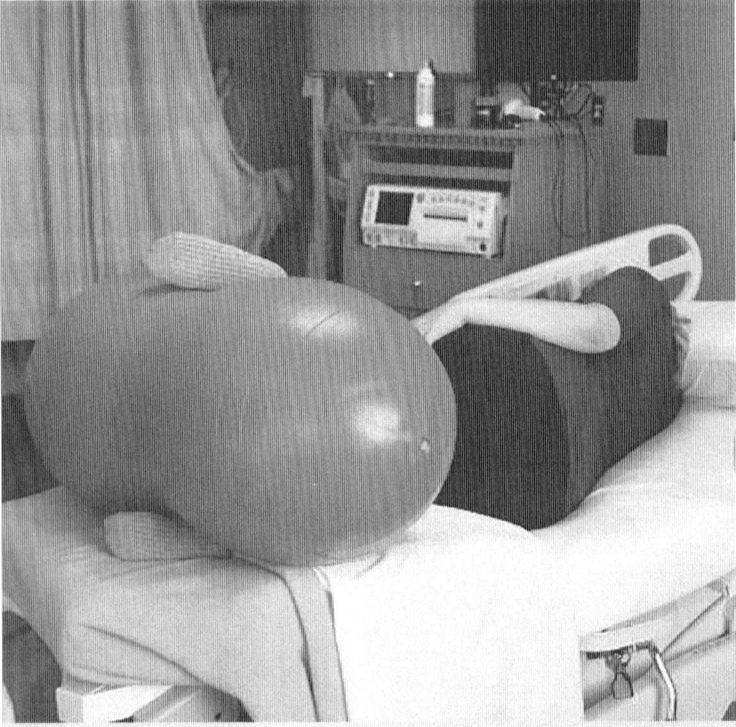

Knees together, Side-Lying, towel between knees. Sitz bones opens for baby head. Low Walchers arch bend opens brim *Photos © Premier Birth Tools LLC*

Side-Lying Foot in Stirrup with Peanut Ball

By Sarah Lavonne, RN, Bundle Birth

This position opens the outlet for resting. While lying on one side, one foot rests on the stirrup in Knees Together, Heels Out Position—popularized in the U.S by Spinning Babies® Approved Trainers—and the arms rest on the peanut ball. The knee can be adjusted based on the location of the baby. Just be sure to support the knee, especially if the client has had an epidural. You can also adjust the foot of bed lower or higher, so as to not overstrain the hip joints.

- Lying on one side, one-foot rests on the stirrup in a knee-to-knee position
- Arms rest on the peanut ball. Use the correct size of peanut ball for comfort
- Adjust the foot of bed lower or higher, so as to not overstrain the hip joints. Use the correct size of peanut ball for comfort

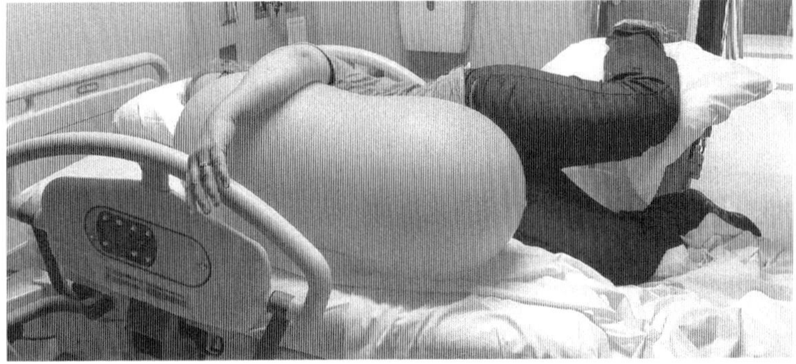

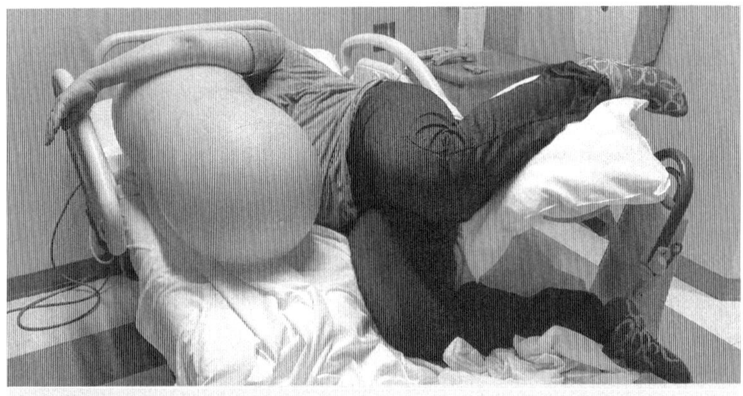

Photos © courtesy of Amy Emerson, RN, Doula for Birth

The "W" Position

By Sarah Lavonne, RN, Bundle Birth

This position combines two peanut ball positions: opens outlet for Resting Hands and Knees Position and the Knees Together Heels Out, popularized in the U.S. by Spinning Babies® Approved Trainers. Then place the client's feet on pillows in the stirrups. This provides support, as well as a stretch to open the outlet. With an epidural, you can use the handlebars padded with pillows. Client can also press the bottom of feet in the foot pedals, or even handle bars padded with pillows, to give some resistance for pushing.

- Place the client's feet on pillows in the stirrups
- Can use the handlebars padded with pillows
- Client can press bottom of feet in the foot pedals or handle bars padded with pillows to give some resistance for pushing

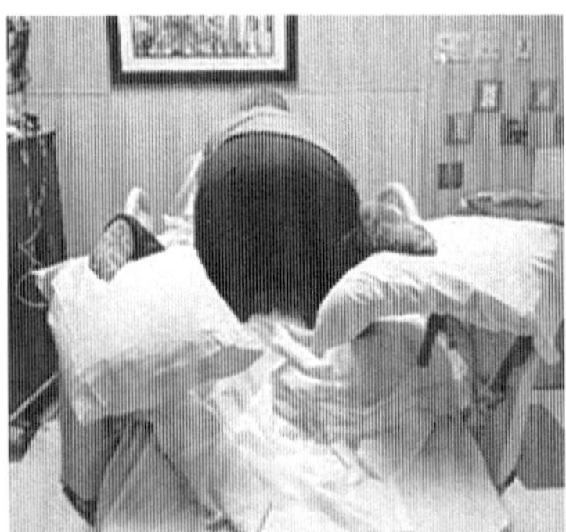

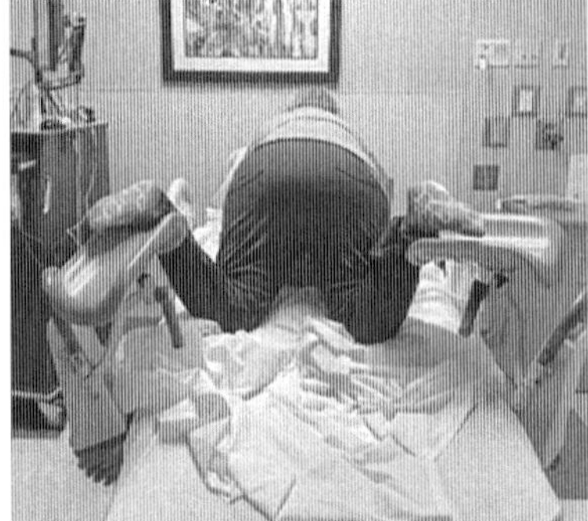

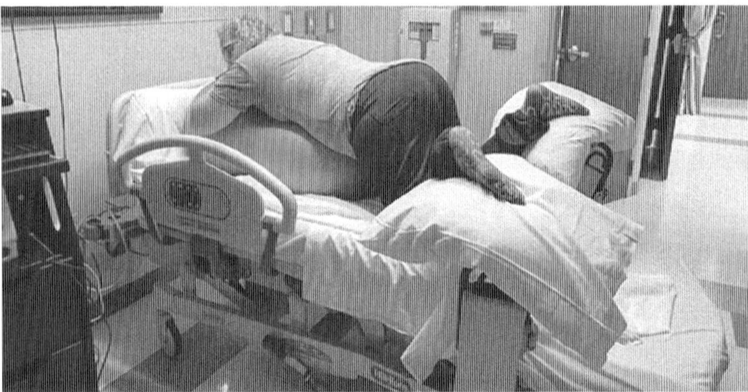

Photos © courtesy of Amy Emerson, RN, Doula for Birth

Semi-Sitting Lunge with Peanut Ball Knee to Knee

By Sarah Lavonne, RN, Bundle Birth

This position opens the outlet for resting and combines two peanut ball positions. The Semi-Sitting Lunge is by Cheri Grant, RN. Make sure the knee is pointed inward like the Knees Together Heels Out, popularized in the U.S. by Spinning Babies® Approved Trainers.

- Sit client up, tilted on their side
- Place top leg over the peanut ball
- Knee is pointed inward, same as the Knee to Knee Position
- Can rock peanut ball back and forth if the baby is mispositioned

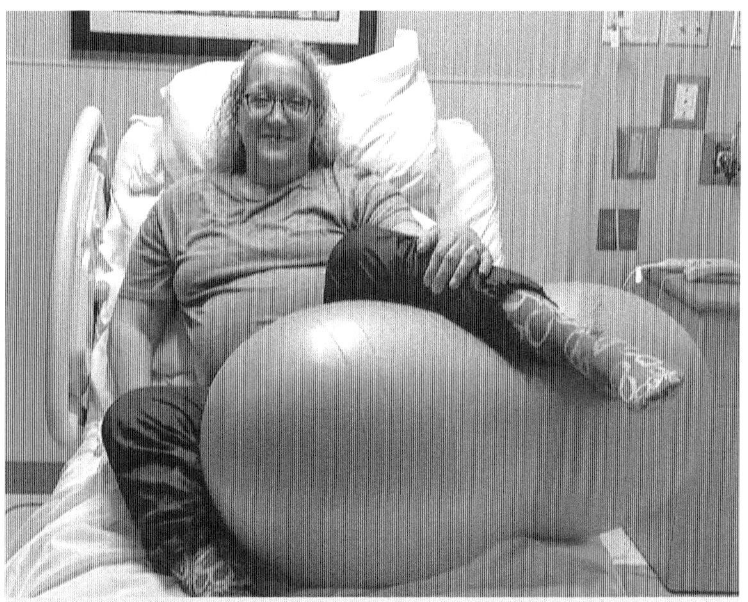

Photo © courtesy of Amy Emerson, RN, Doula for Birth

Learn More

Check out Sarah Lavonne, RN, Bundle Birth, A Nursing Corporation website to learn more: bundlebirth.com

Yes! We're all in it together, here to work together for the betterment of birthing families! Love it when nurses get creative!

Sarah Lavonne, RN, Bundle Birth, A Nursing Coporation

Facilitate Internal Rotation of Femur or Thigh Bone

By Amy Bookwalter, CD

To assist internal rotation, place the leg on the peanut ball with a rolled towel under the top ankle. This allows knee to knee and opens the outlet.

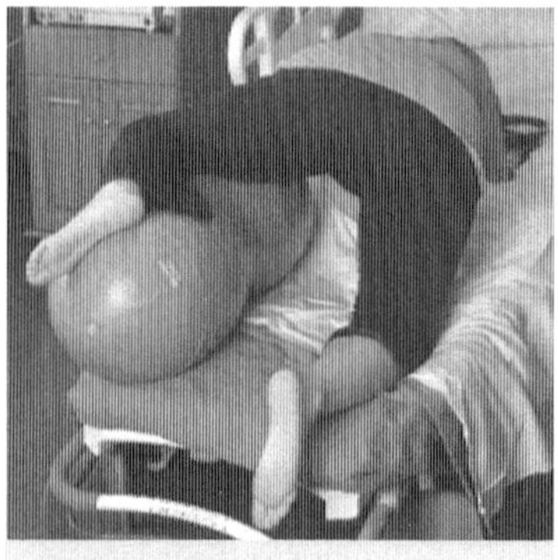

Photo © Premier Birth Tools LLC

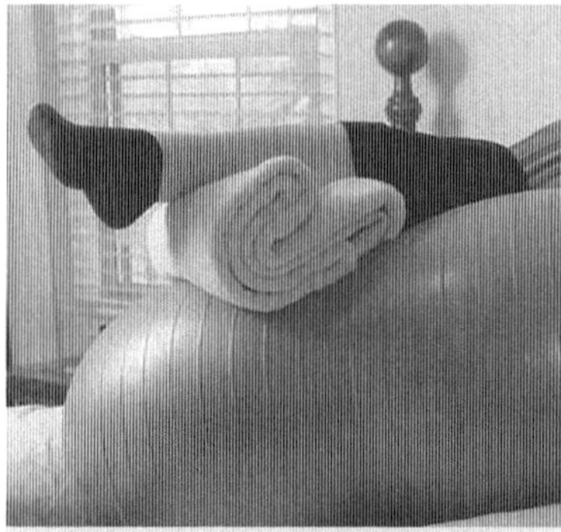

Photos © courtesy of Amy Bookwalter, CD

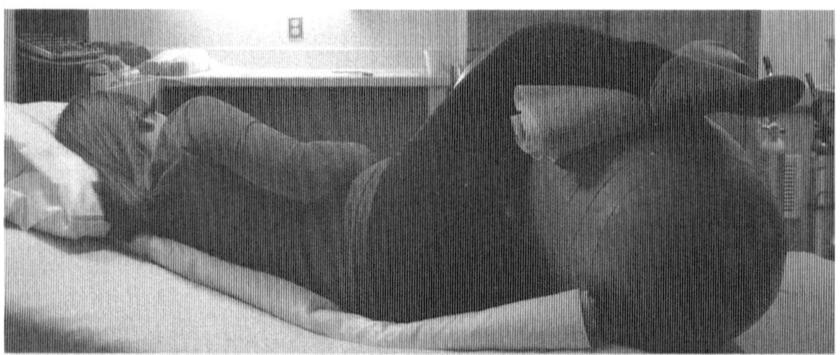

Internal rotation of femur or thigh bone; baby low in pelvis, below +1 station. *Photo © courtesy Photos by Amy Bookwalter, CD*

Sitting with Legs on Peanut Ball

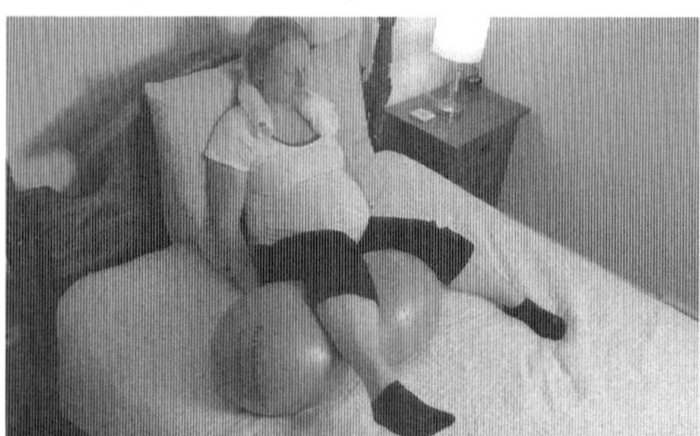

Outlet internal rotation of femur or thigh bones. *Photo courtesy Amy Bookwalter, CD*

I have used the peanut ball many times and I am a huge advocate for them, especially while resting with an epidural. One time that I can remember the peanut ball helping someone avoid a Cesarean, was a client with an epidural and baby was having decels. I had a feeling it was due to compression, because the baby was moving into the outlet and didn't have much space. I suggested Side-Lying [Position] with the peanut ball placed between ankles, knees together (internal rotation) to open the outlet, and my client was able to rest. Decels stopped altogether and transition happened almost immediately. The baby was born shortly after . . . and the staff was amazed.

Nicole Sawyers Todd, doula, Pennsylvania

OTHER OUTLET POSITIONS

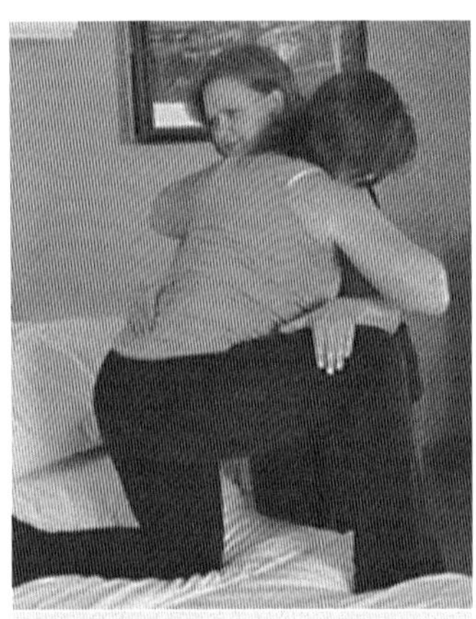

Lunge to side.
Kneel on one leg with foot flat, and diagonal to pelvis.

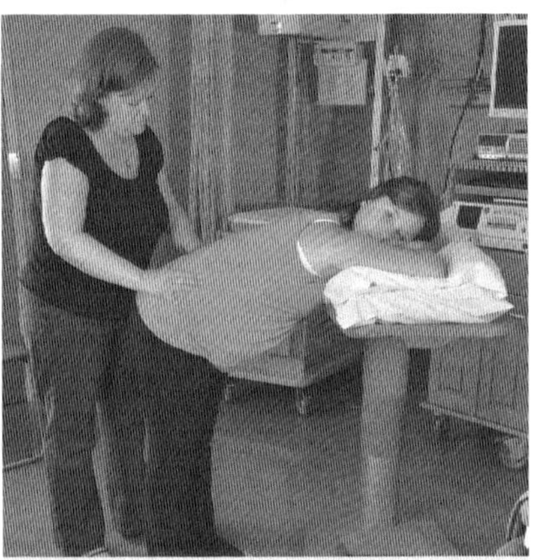

Stand, holding something higher than belly. Bend knees, stand with heels turned out and toes turned in.

Outlet—Baby Out

Internal rotation of femur thigh bones =

Outlet = Get baby out

Internal rotation opens BOTTOM of pelvis

Knees together pointing inward= Knee to knee

Knees in, heels out, and toes turned in pointing together

Knees pointing in—Opens outlet—BOTTOM of pelvis

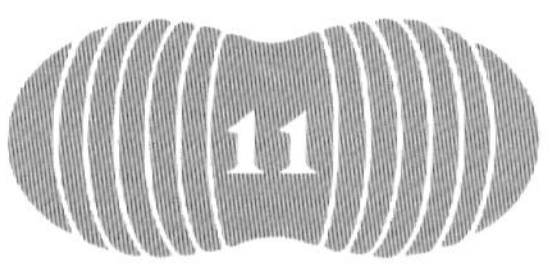

USING A PEANUT BALL WITH AN EPIDURAL

"As a doula, I have had many mothers who are in active labor and want to lay on their side, with or without an epidural. The peanut ball is just what they need to open their pelvis and allow the baby to come down while still resting. I have seen it help mothers quickly progress many times—even in times of stress where the care provider gives a time clock of X hours to be fully dilated or give birth or threatens to do a Cesarean section. I am amazed at how it helps women progress and reduces second-stage length. I would not be on-call for a labor without it and I love sharing it with all of my birth-worker friends!"

—Bethany Stricker, doula and
Peanut Ball Ambassador, Texas

MANY OF THE POSITIONS shared in this book can also be used if the client has an epidural. One of the great advantages of peanut ball use is that many positions can be used while the patient is in bed. Its use truly facilitates labor progression. So many mothers can avoid Cesarean Delivery with the use of motion changes, facilitated by peanut ball positions.

One should make sure to have extra help and support when transitioning to each new peanut ball position. Support the limbs and do not twist the body when turning. Use caution in positioning, clients may not recognize if they are overstretching, which can lead to injuries or pain after the epidural is gone. It is also important to understand the internal and external rotation of the femur or thigh bone discussed earlier, and pay attention to which way the femur or thigh bone is rotated. (These positions have been described in depth in other chapters of this book, so only titles will be listed here.) This is only a few of the postions to use with an epidual. There are many more postions throughout this book.

Side-Lying

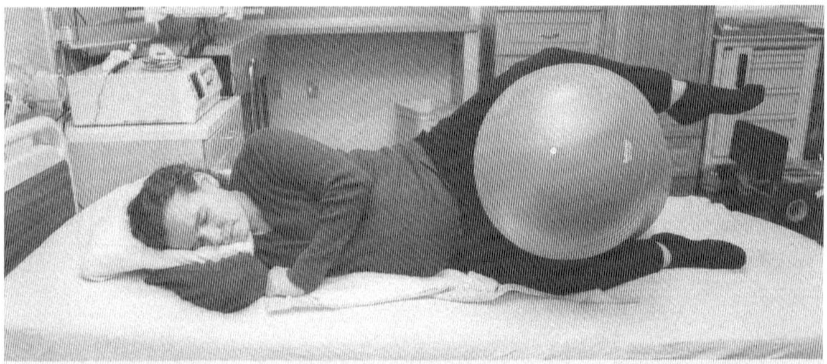

Switching side every 30 minutes to an hour. *Photo courtesy of Amy Bookwalter, CD*

Tuck Position

By Cheri Grant, RN, Premier Birth Tools

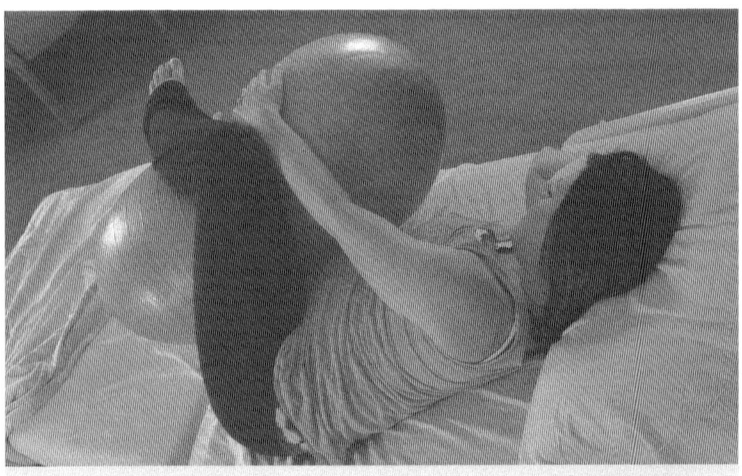

Pull both knees up to chest. *Photos © Premier Birth Tools LLC*

Rock the Boat

By Tammy Ryan, SpBT

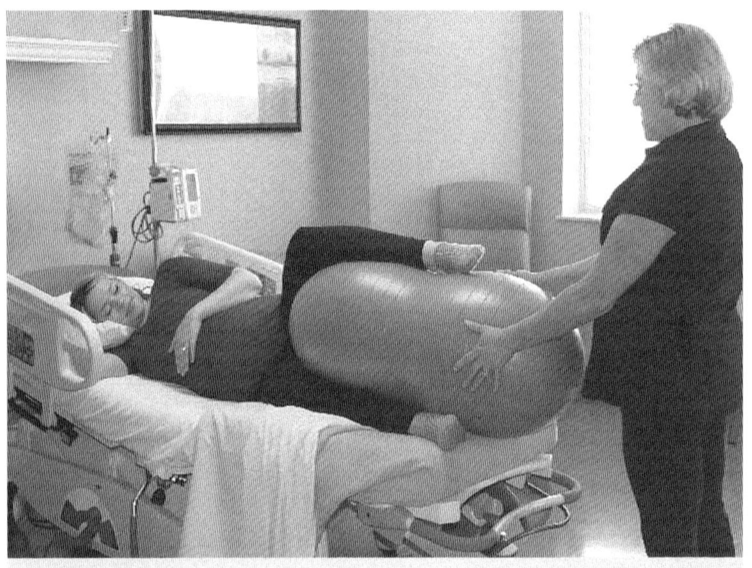

Maintain movement of the pelvis.

Note: *See Chapter 9 for detailed information on this position.*

Flying Cowgirl

By Gail Tully, CPM, Spinning Babies®

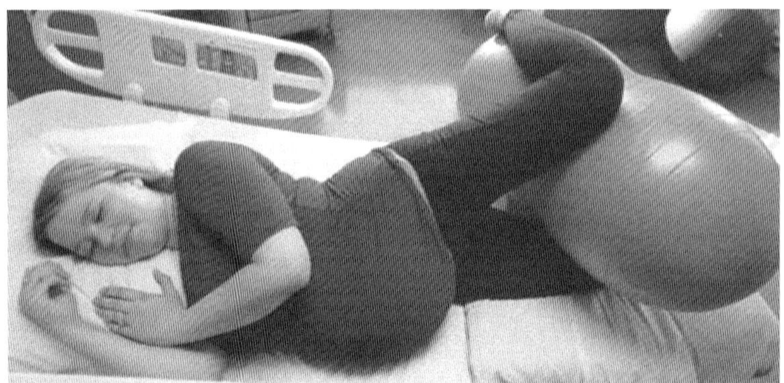

Knee bending back and behind hip or pelvis. *Photos © Premier Birth Tools LLC*

Note: *See Chapter 8 for detailed information on this position.*

I have worked with several clients. The most recent I was assisting at the birth center. The client was 2-3 cm. Mostly effaced. She had her baby within an hour and a half, after doing a Side-Lying Position. One leg over the peanut ball, rocking her hips. It's a position called Rocking the Boat, [which] Spinning Babies® has recommended. I listened to Cheri Grant, RN, on a podcast on peanut balls and learned new techniques that I used during this birth.

Joanna Zepeda, Doula and Dancing for Birth Instructor, Texas

"Rollover Sequence" with an Epidural

By Penny Simkin PT

This Rollover Sequence technique was introduced in the 1990s, by Penny Simkin, PT, for use with an epidural. It is for use when there is no indication of malposition or when it is difficult to determine the location of the fetal back. It is wonderful to use with an epidural and immobility is an issue to increase contractions (Simkin, 2017, 293).

I have modified this to use with peanut balls. Place the client in each position, for 20 to 30 minutes, in the order of the following sequence: Semi-Sitting Lunge, Side-Lying Lunge, Leaning Forward, Side-Lying Lunge, Flying Cowgirl, Knees Together Heels Out, and back to Semi-Sitting Lunge. Penny's original sequence is as follows: Semi-Sitting, left Side-Lying, left Semi-Prone, Hands and Knees, right Semi-Prone, right Side-Lying, and back to Semi-Sitting.

The peanut ball has been a fantastic advent to the care and management of laboring individuals. A multitude of positions can be offered to assist the laborer to minimize discomfort, shorten labor, and avoid a mechanical or surgical delivery, especially when mobility is limited by epidural analgesia.

Dr. Jennifer Klump, DNP, CNM, RN, and Authorized Peanut Ball Trainer, Illinois

Roll Over for Epidural Movement

By Penny Simkin, PT, modified By Cheri Grant, using the peanut ball

Semi-Sitting Lunge—Inlet

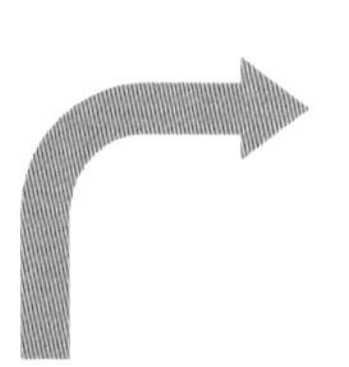

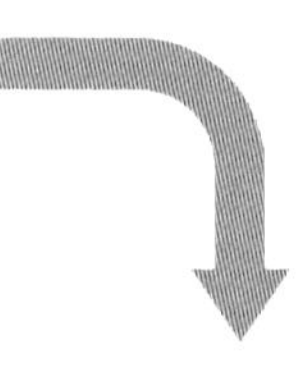

Knees Together, Heels Out—Outlet
Popularized by U.S. Spinning Babies® Approved Trainers

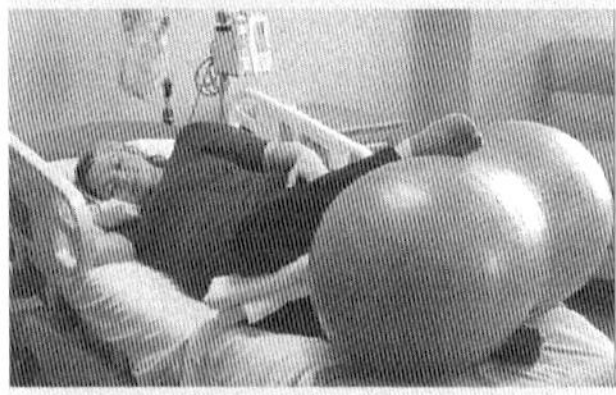

Knees together, side lying. Towel between knees.

Flying Cowgirl—Knees Outward—Inlet
By Gail Tully, CPM, Spinning Babies®

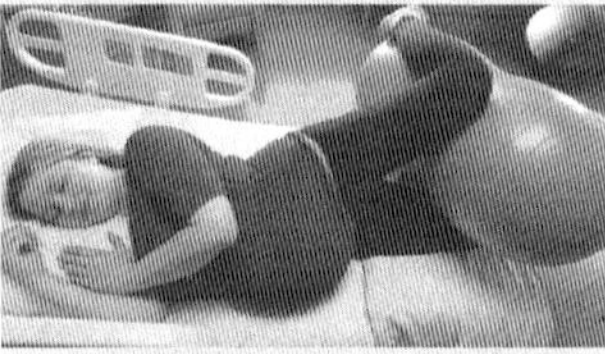

Knee behind hip. Pelvis tucked open inlet -2 external rotation femur

Side-Lying Runners—Midpelvis, knees parallel

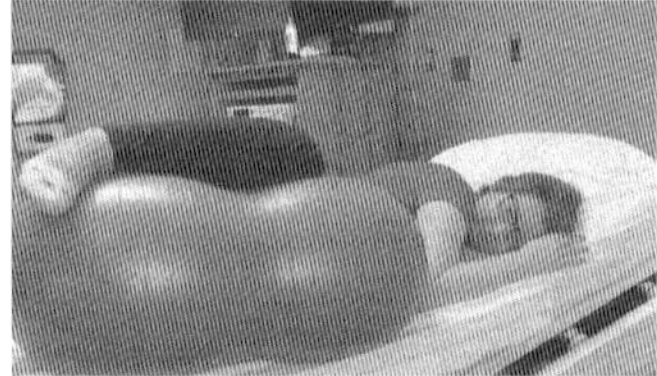

Upper body rotate, chest facing down on bed on stomach. Back hand behind.

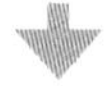

Leaning Forward

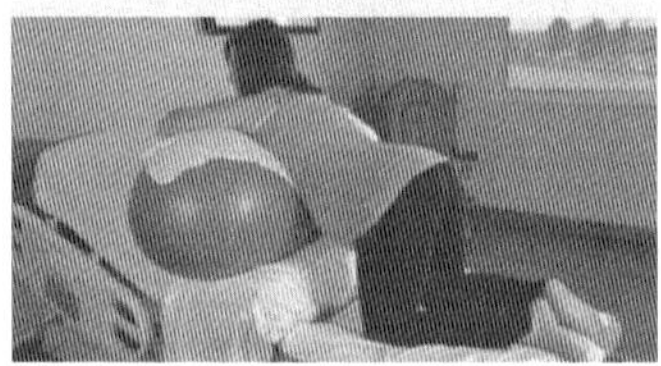

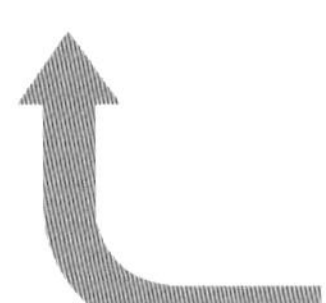

Side-Lying Lunge—Midpelvis

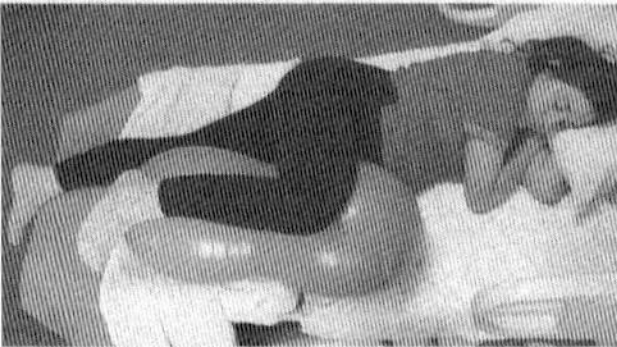

Baby moves *up*. Reposition head and tuck chin. Bottom leg straight. Peanut ball in front.

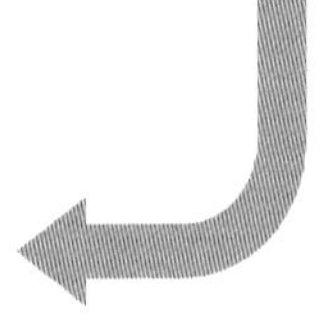

"Patient was at 5 cm/-1 station for several hours. The operating room was notified of a possible Cesarean section. I came on [my] shift to find my patient with an epidural and a pillow between her knees (which had slipped away) and her pelvis very closed. I helped her use a peanut ball for 30 minutes on one side, which allowed a lower station for AROM. Then we used the peanut ball left [side for] 30 minutes, right [side for] 30 minutes, and delivery occurred two to three hours after AROM!"

Nicole Page, nurse, Indiana

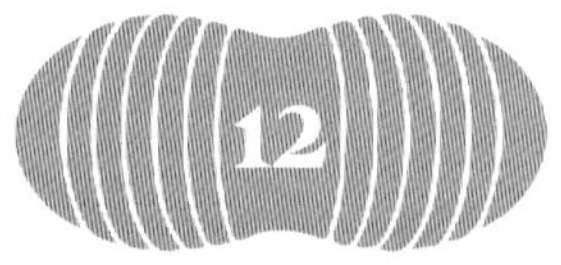

PUSHING WITH THE PEANUT BALL

"Our first time using the peanut ball, several years ago, the OB physician, (who for the most part is very hesitant to change routines or try new ideas) made fun of us and the whole concept. That patient then delivered a 10 -pound, 4-ounce baby after using it in [the] second stage of labor. Now, *he insists we use it on every labor patient of his."*

—Darlene McClimans, nurse, and Authorized Peanut Ball Trainer Illinios

PUSHING WITH A PEANUT BALL is possible and is typically more comfortable than when using stirrups. It can be done with an epidural too! Peanut balls have also been shown to reduce the pushing phase of labor by an average of 22 minutes (Tussy, 2011).

Pushing with a Peanut Ball Versus the Stirrup—Opens Outlet Wider

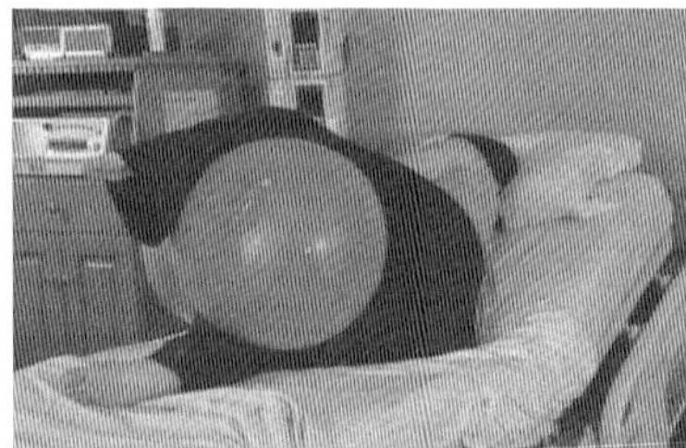

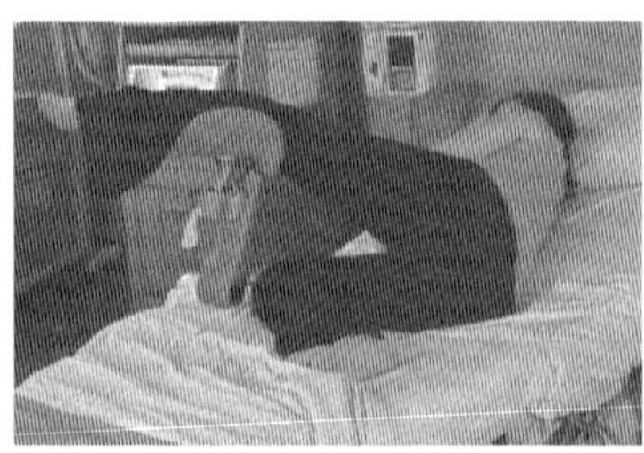

Photos © Premier Birth Tools LLC

Tuck Position

By Cheri Grant, RN, Premier Birth Tools

The Tuck Position opens the outlet and is like squatting. The provider still has a full view of perineum in this position.

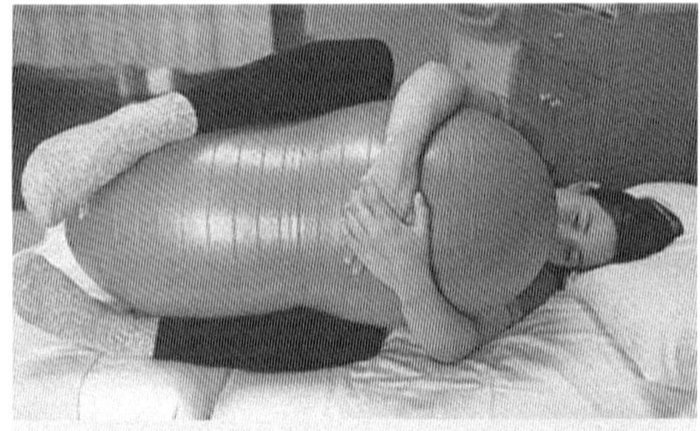

Photo © Premier Birth Tools LLC

> *The physicians now request the peanut ball after seeing how it helps shorten the second stage!*
>
> **Kathryn Fauver, A Childbirth Educator and Peanut Ball Ambassador from Illinois**

Tuck and Pull

By Mandy Irby, RN, "The Birth Nurse"

This position was invented by Mandy Irby, RN, and Authorized Peanut Ball Trainer. She us also known as "The Birth Nurse" (Irby, 2019 video).

- Wrap a sheet around the back of the bar at the head of birthing bed
- Then tuck and pull

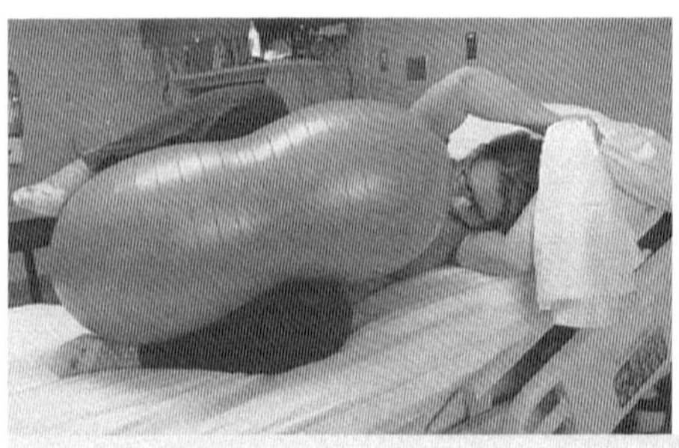

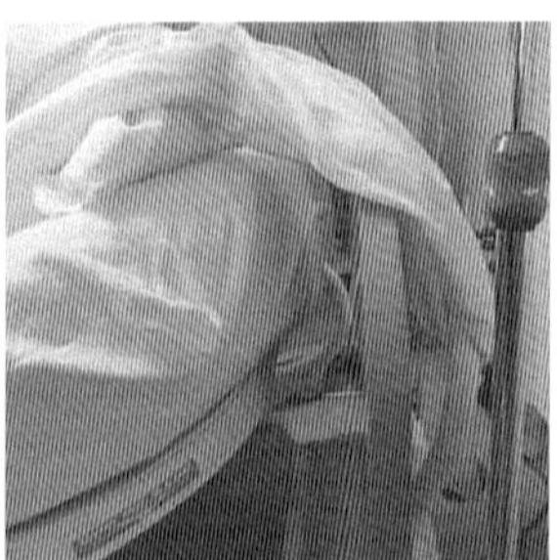

Photos © Premier Birth Tools LLC

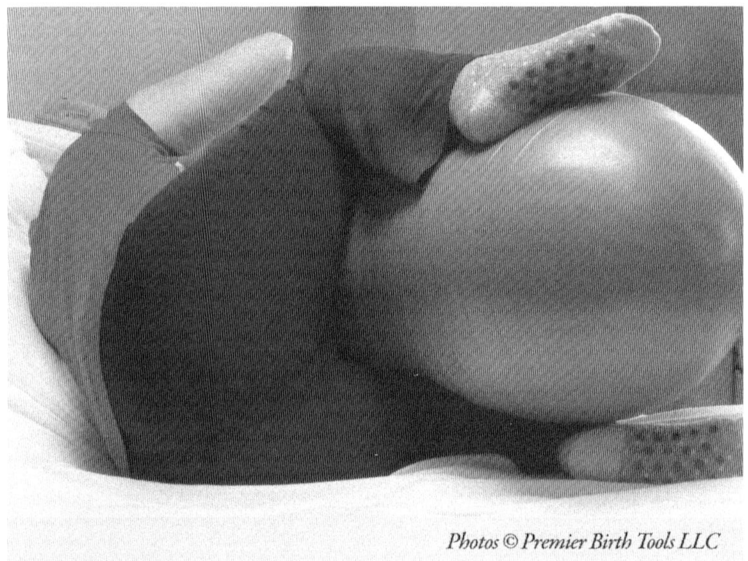

Photos © Premier Birth Tools LLC

Mandy Irby, RN, The Birth Nurse, teaches an excellent online peanut ball class. This Birth Nurse workshop includes, "Peanut Balls in Labor: Beginner and Advanced Skills for Labor Nurses and Doulas."

Learn More

Visit The Birth Nurse website to learn more: mandyirby.com

> *Peanut balls are some of the most powerful tools in a Labor and Delivery nurse's tool kit. They facilitate labor and trust at the same time!*
>
> Mandy Irby, nurse and Authorized Peanut Ball Trainer

Hands and Knees Pushing

Pushing on Hands and Knees supported with a peanut ball is an excellent pushing position. *See Chapter 10 for detailed information on this position.*

Extreme Tuck Pushing

This position is different from the Tuck, as the tuck movement is more towards client's chest. This position maintains the wide-open posture needed for pushing without exerting energy. It also gives the provider full view of the perineum and maintains a true Side-Lying Position.

Note: *It may be difficult to monitor the client in this position.*

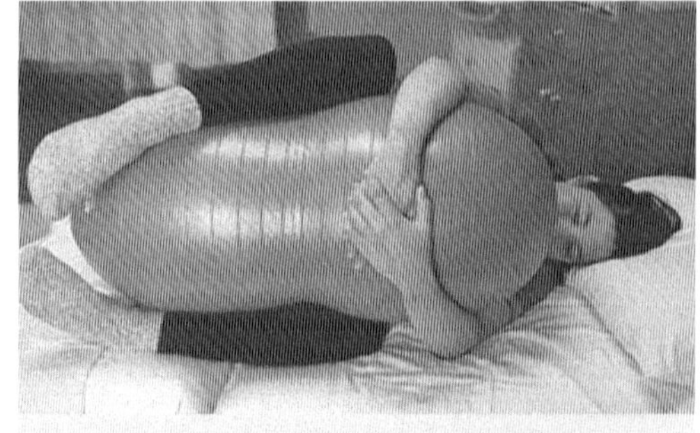

Photo © Premier Birth Tools LLC

- Tuck is toward chest
- In Side-Lying Position, hug peanut ball while pushing

I use the peanut ball often to get baby to descend down, then to get baby to get crowning.

Sheradawn Sullivan, nurse, Idaho

Hip Tilt Tuck Pushing

Client is in Tuck Postion, but also tilts the pelvis.

"Peanut ball I prefer calling it the birth bullet! Stated a very happy client, using the peanut ball during labor and birth!"

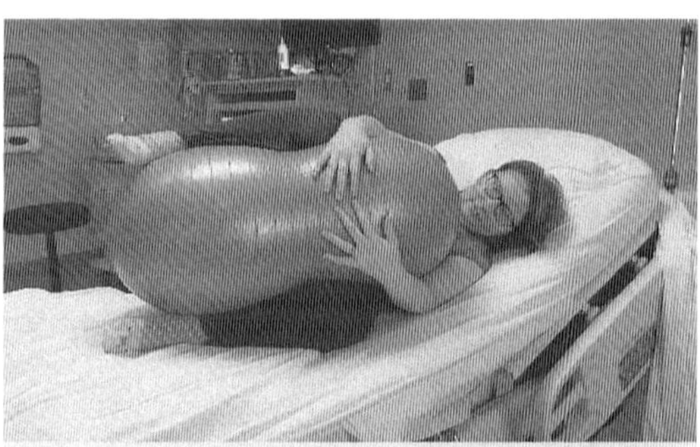

Photo © Premier Birth Tools LLC

Lunge Curl Pushing

By Mandy Irby, RN, The Birth Nurse

Mandy introduced this position in her "Pushing with Peanut Ball" video (Irby, 2019, video).

- Bring the ball to the chest
- Hang leg straight over the ball

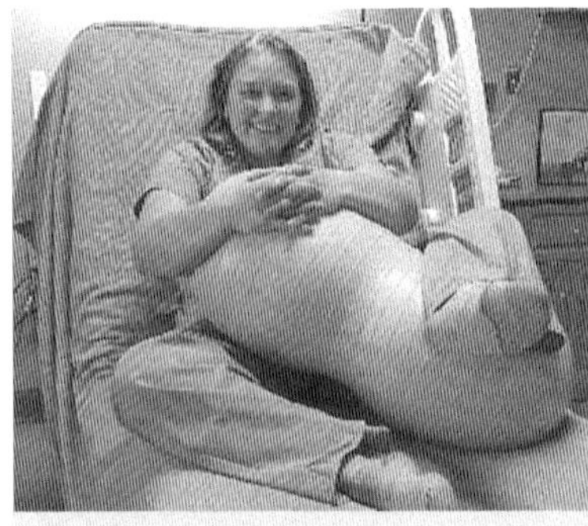

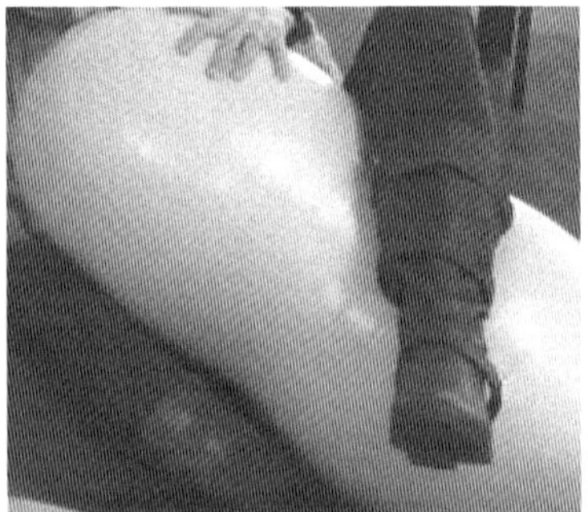

Photos © Premier Birth Tools LLC

Asymmetrical Kneeling for Pushing

By Heidi Duncan, CBD (CBI)

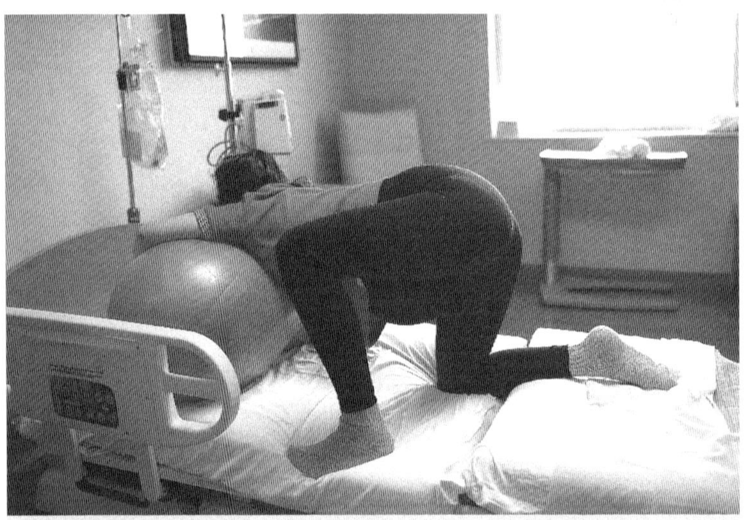

If client rotates both ankles out it opens the bottom of pelvis more. *Photo © Premier Birth Tools LLC*

In the Asymmetrical Kneeling for Pushing Posistion, face the end of the bed and use a squat bar, if available, on the bed. Then place the client in a Kneeling Asymmetrical Position for pushing during second stage. Slide the peanut ball under the elevated leg during breaks to allow a shift of weight and to rest. This is more sustainable than Squatting for many clients. The ball can be removed when delivering the baby and the client can easily catch her baby in this position. If the client is kneeling facing the foot of the bed, they can easily transition to Side-Lying Position, if desired, rather than lying directly on their back as typically happens when moving from a squatting position in the bed. If they are facing the head of the bed, they can move to their hands and knees.

- Place squat bar on the bed
- Place client in a Kneeling Asymmetrical Position for pushing
- Slide peanut ball under the elevated leg during breaks to allow a shift of weight and rest
- Ball can be removed when delivering the baby

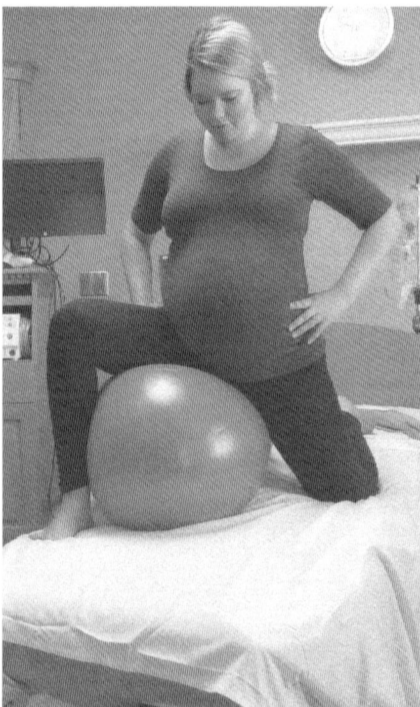

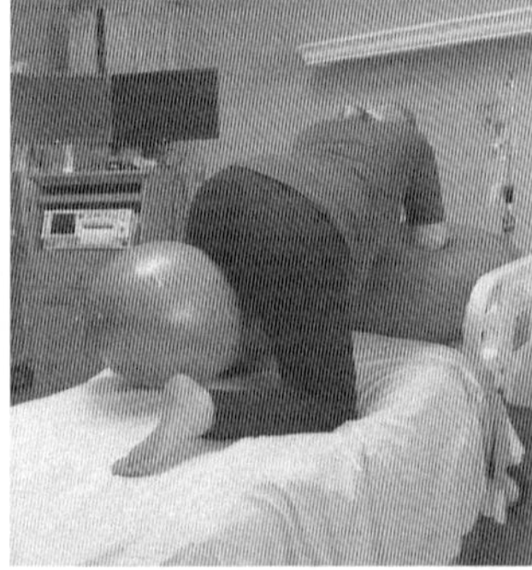

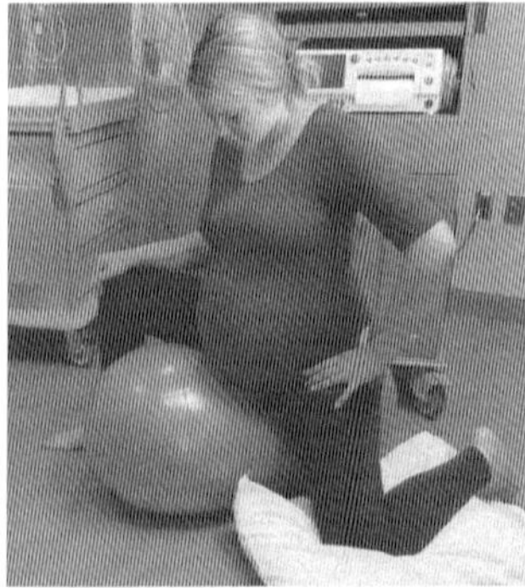

Photos © Premier Birth Tools LLC

Knees Together Pushing: Heels Out

Popularized in the US by Spinning Babies® Approved Trainers

Internal rotation of the femur or thigh bone, applied for birth with knees together and heels out, is demonstrated in *Preparing for a Gentle Birth: The Pelvis in Pregnancy* by authors Blandine Callais Germain and Núria Vives Parés (German and Parés, 2012). I highly recommend this book as supplemental reading. Commonly called Knees-Together Pushing Position, this position is used during the contraction when baby is low in the pelvis. Turning the toes toward each other rotates the thigh bone to widen the sitz bones. This position was popularized in the U.S. by Spinning Babies® Approved Trainers. *See Chapter 10 for detailed information about this position*

- Knees are together with heels apart and toes pointing to each other
- Peanut ball between ankle
- Keeping knees together, pull them up towards the chest to push with heels out

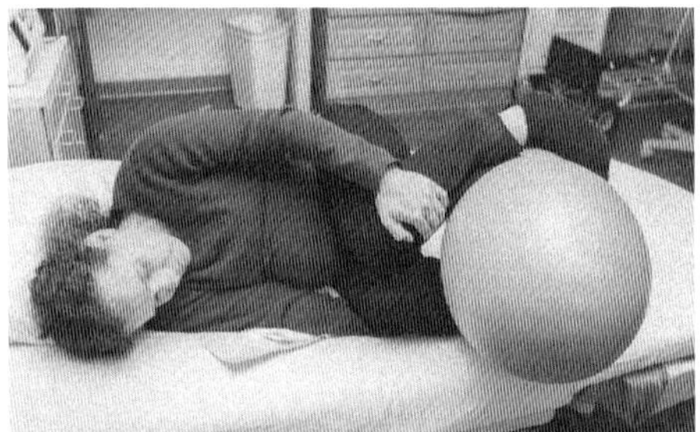

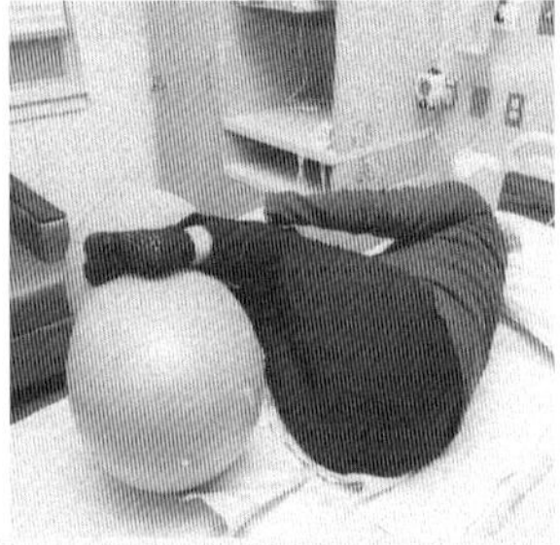

Knees Together Pushing: Heels Out - Internal rotation of femur .

Photo courtesy Amy Bookwalter, CD

PEANUT BALL PUSHING VIDEOS

Knees Together Pushing Video

This video does a great job of demonstrating opening the bottom of the pelvis for pushing outlet opening. Visit MamasteFit Training on YouTube for this video: "Opening the Bottom of the Pelvis for Pushing" (Outlet Opening, 2019).

Another Great Video

Visit Lamaze.org, Connecting the Dots blog post (Cockeram, Mindy, 2020), "Narrow the Knees to Push with Ease: Challenge The Norm and Get The Job Done!"

Peanut Ball Pushing Video

By Mandy Irby, RN

Visit Mandy Irby's YouTube channel and look for the video titled "What Does It Look Like to Push with Peanut Balls?" (Peanut Balls in Labor, 2019).

PEANUT BALL PUSHING POSITIONS CHART

We offer Peanut Ball Pushing Positions Charts at Premier Birth Tools. This packet includes 11 pushing positions with 26 pictures, including positions with and without the epidural. Find out more by visiting the store on premierbirthtools.com

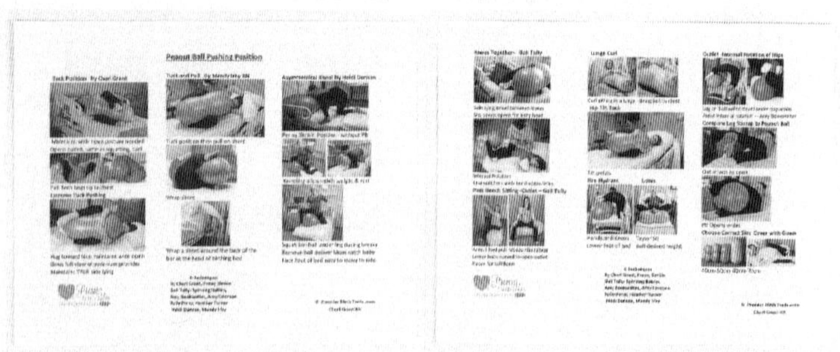

> *Your charts are amazing and I cannot wait for our staff at my hospital to use them!*
>
> Lori Putnick, nurse, Virginia

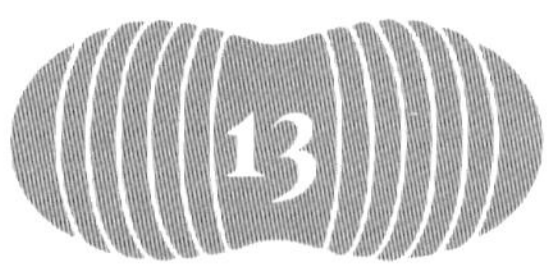

ASYMMETRICAL VARIATIONS USING THE PEANUT BALL

"Peanut ball is amazing! I've been a labor and delivery nurse for 18 years and I am now a manager. I love using them and see their implications for practice!"

—Tabby Bonner, nurse, Georgia

ASYMMETRICAL POSITIONS HELP facilitate and enhance the rotation of the femur or thigh bone, as the baby enters the pelvis. Most asymmetrical peanut ball positions are used for midpelvis. *See Chapter 9 for more information.*

Asymmetrical Kneeling

This position can be done while seated on the ball for support. It will encourage the baby to rotate into an easier position for labor and birth. Comfort guides the client as to which leg to raise. *See Chapter 12 for more information.*

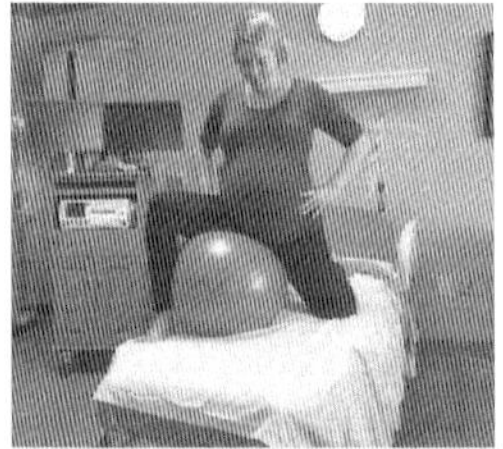

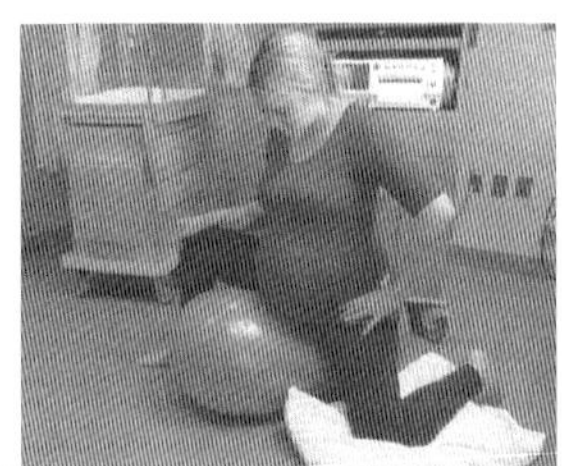

Photos © Premier Birth Tools LLC

Asymmetrical Sitting

This position encourages the baby to rotate into an easier position for labor and birth.

- Elevate the head of the bed
- Hang one leg over the indentation of peanut ball and the other leg over bed

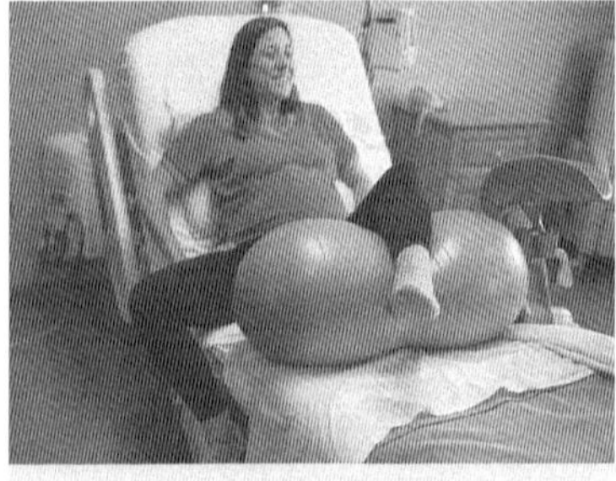

Leg hangs off the bed.
Photo © Premier Birth Tools LLC

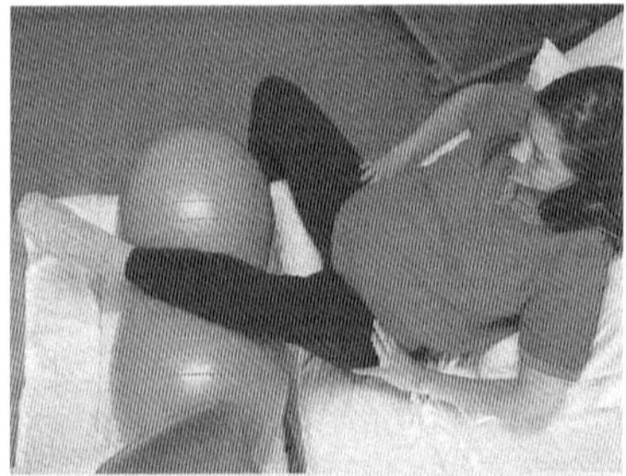

Careful of client's position.
Photo © Premier Birth Tools LLC

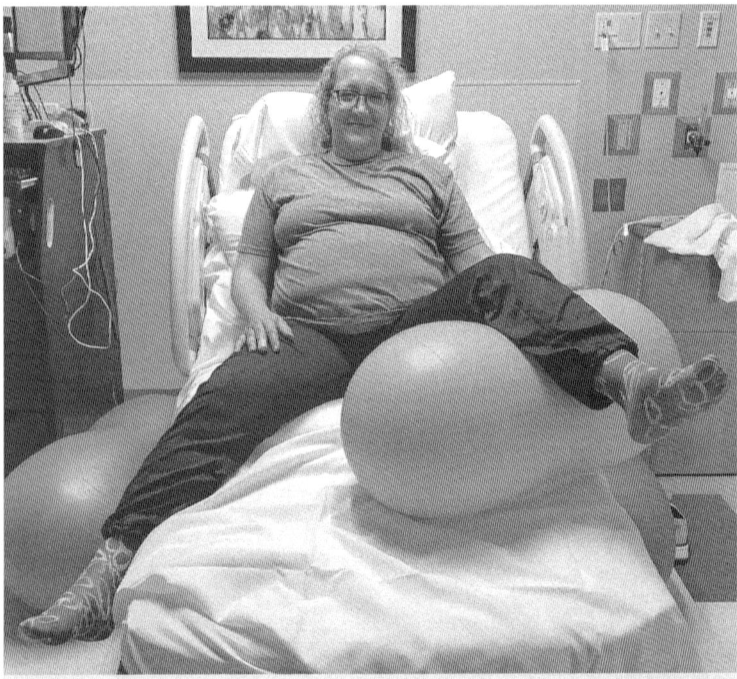

Photo courtesy of Amy Emerson, RN

Asymmetrical Kneel Position

By Heidi Duncan, CBD (CBI)

Comfort guides the client as to which leg they will raise. The more comfortable side is the side the client should use. *See Chapter 12 for more information.*

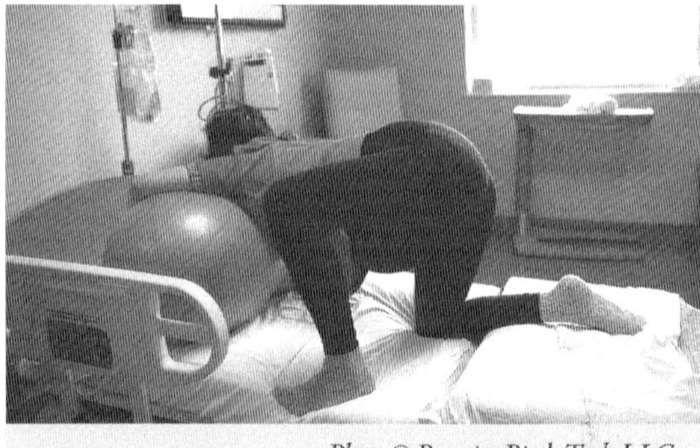

Photo © Premier Birth Tools LLC

Hands and Knees, Kneeling and Straddling

This position requires two peanut balls. Place client on their hands and knees. Have them straddle one peanut ball and lean forward onto a smaller peanut ball. Be aware that in this position, the back-end of the peanut ball may want to pop up. To avoid this, keep a hand pressing down towards the bed on the back-end of the ball. You can also use a sheet to tie that end of the peanut ball to the bed.

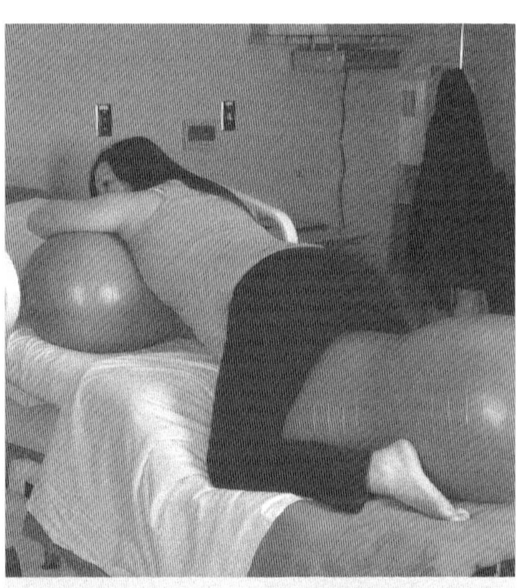

Photo © Premier Birth Tools LLC

- Place client on hands and knees and lower the bottom of the bed
- Have client and lean forward onto a smaller peanut ball
- Straddle peanut ball; use only hospital grade to sit on

Standing Asymmetrical Kneeling Over Peanut Ball

Adjust the height of the bed for the client. Have them stand beside bed, kneeling on it and leaning over the peanut ball.

- Adjust the height of the bed for the client
- Stand beside bed
- Kneel on the bed and lean over the peanut ball

In *The Labor Progress Handbook* (2017) by Penny Simkin, Lisa Hansen, and Ruth Anceta, discusses this position and many others. I have modified many of the positions discussed in Penny's book to use with a peanut ball. I highly recommend Penny's book as supplemental reading.

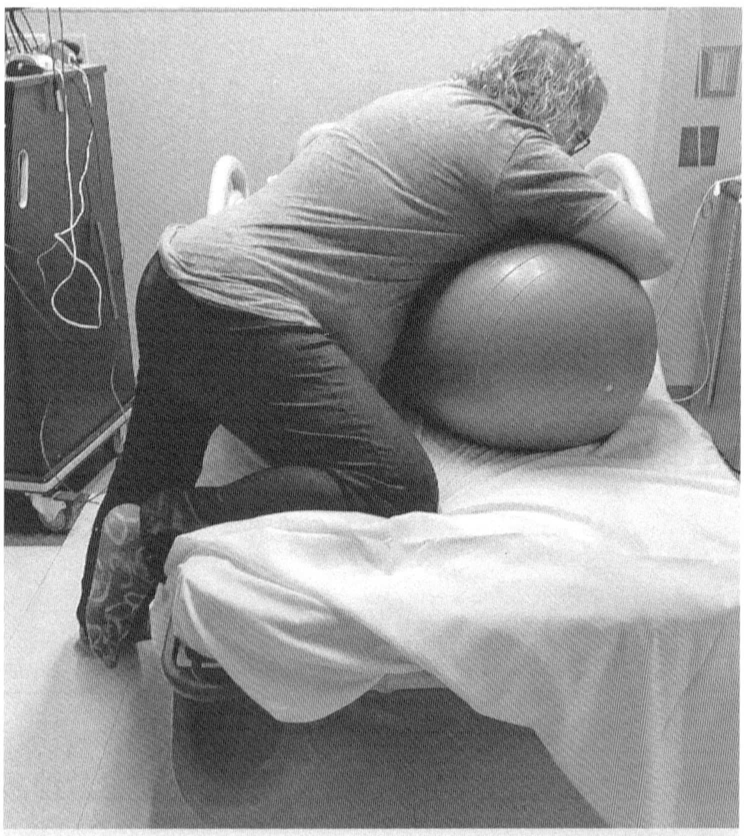

Photo courtesy of Amy Emerson, RN, Doula for Birth

I have watched a lot of my doula clients make amazing progress using the peanut ball. The most vivid memory I have with a client was hearing the nurse state that they wanted [the] mom to try pushing to see if she could "get anywhere'"and then they would talk about Cesarean section once she was around 24-hours beyond [her] water breaking. The nurse told the mom that 'sometimes babies just don't come out and I don't think this one is going to," before telling us she'd give us an hour to "try whatever we'd like." I assisted her in doing a circuit of 20 minutes Side-Lying with [the] peanut ball; 20 minutes Tailor Sitting, doing hip circles, while leaning over the peanut ball; and then 20 minutes Side-Lying on the opposite side. When the nurse came back in to do a cervical check before contacting the doctor to book the operating room, she was absolutely shocked that mom was fully dilated and [the] baby had descended. She was ready to push and [the] baby was born vaginally. Mom was using an epidural in this case. It was one of the few times I truly felt my assistance actively played a large role in helping a mom avoid a Cesarean section. This wouldn't have been possible without the peanut ball.

Christy High, childbirth educator, Kentucky

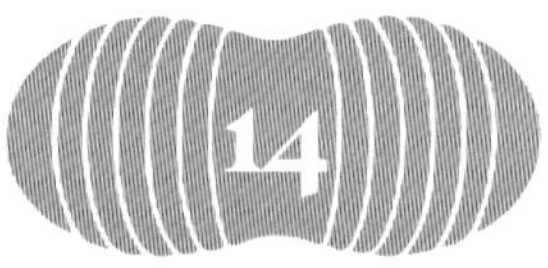

PEANUT BALL BREECH TILT

"Breech is my passion. Most of my 10 pregnancies have been breech. I delivered two of my breeches vaginally with great medical support. Most moms don't have this option, so I work to help countless other moms to find room to flip their babies during pregnancy."

—Rebekah Porter, doula and Peanut Ball Ambassador, Tennessee

PEANUT BALLS CAN BE USED in the Breech Tilt Position to help a baby find room to turn. It can be a difficult position to hold, but it is easier if someone can place the peanut ball under the client's back.

Rebekah Porter, a certified doula, invented this position, while working with clients. When a baby is in breech position prior to labor (34 weeks or later), it is possible to have the baby turn to a head-down position to avoid a Cesarean section. Several positions help, but the one described in this chapter can be used very successfully, during pregnancy and in labor. It is more comfortable and has a higher success rate than following the traditional ironing board idea.

Peanut Ball Breech Tilt Position

By Rebekah Porter, CD, Blissful Birthing

- Have the client lay on the floor, on her back, with her legs resting on a couch or chair
- Then have her push her back up and off the floor, and slide a peanut ball behind her. (A second ball or pillow can be added if needed)
- The client needs to be close to the couch and can grab the peanut ball to pull herself closer if necessary
- Sizing of peanut balls is important in this position, as always

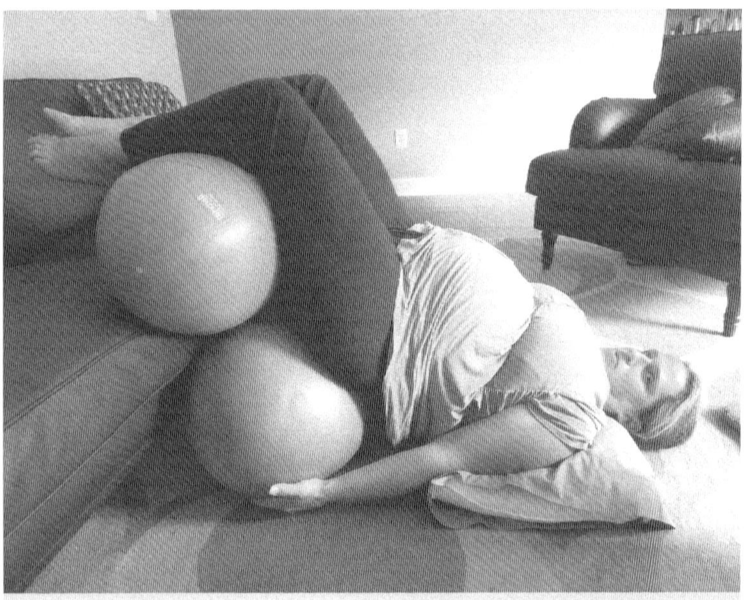

Breech Peanut Ball Tilt. *Photo courtesy of Rebekah Porter*

Learn More

For more information on this position, visit Blissful Birthing where you will find a free download about this position: blissfulbirthingtn.com/post/breech-babies-and-peanut-balls

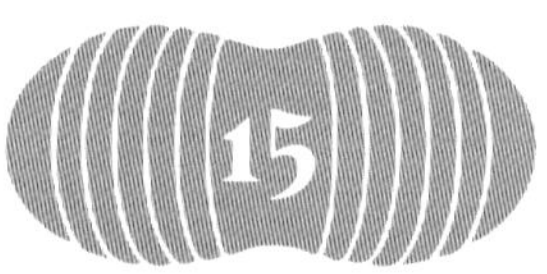

FUN POSITIONS CLIENTS INVENTED DURING LABOR

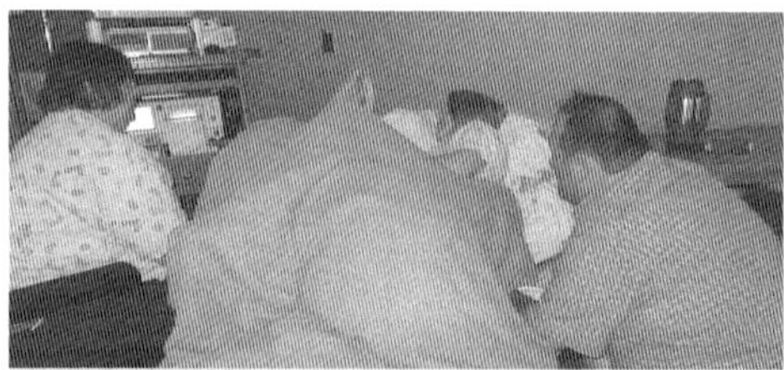

Cheri with a client.
Photo © Premier Birth Tools LLC

"I use peanut balls all the time both in home and out-of-home births. It has been so helpful for lots of mamas."

—Toni Hill, doula, Mississippi

THERE ARE ALREADY SO MANY different peanut ball positions, but it is always fun to see what new peanut ball positions clients invent while in labor. Here are just a few:

Resting Lying on Peanut Ball with Legs Up in Chair

- This position is a combination of Open Knee Chest and Forward Leaning Inversion

- This position allowed the client to be comfortable and also allows the baby to hang
- Ball should be small to align the shoulders lower than the hips
- Place a rolled towel in front and behind the ball to help stabilize the ball

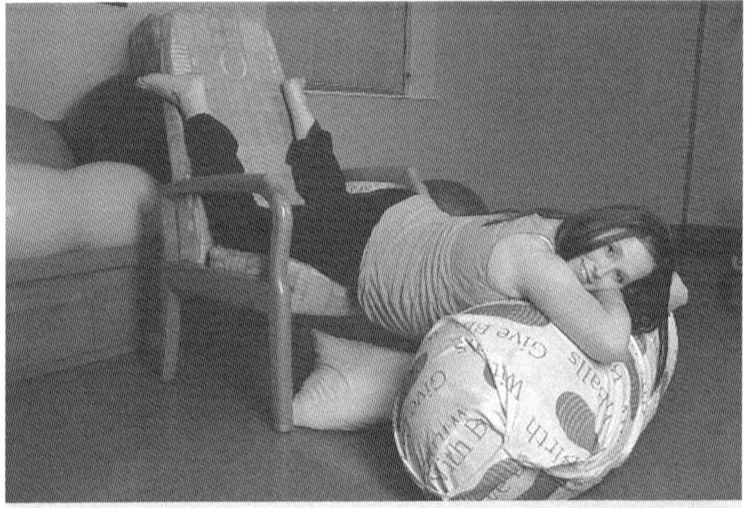

Photo © Premier Birth Tools LLC

Arching Back Lying with Feet on Ball

Client wanted to lie down and put legs up on peanut ball, as client found it felt good in lumbar area to stretch or arch the back.

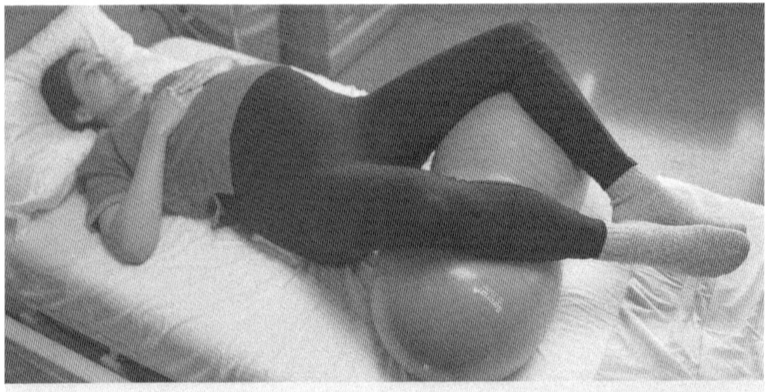

Photo © Premier Birth Tools LLC

Caution: *Not every Peanut Ball position is a good position.*

Semi-Lying with Feet on Ball

Not every peanut ball position is a good position. This client wanted to lie down, but didn't want to be on her hips in a Side-Lying Position. Client wanted to rest with legs up on the peanut ball. Be careful this position might encourage baby to turn occiput posterior or to slow baby's rotation or descent.

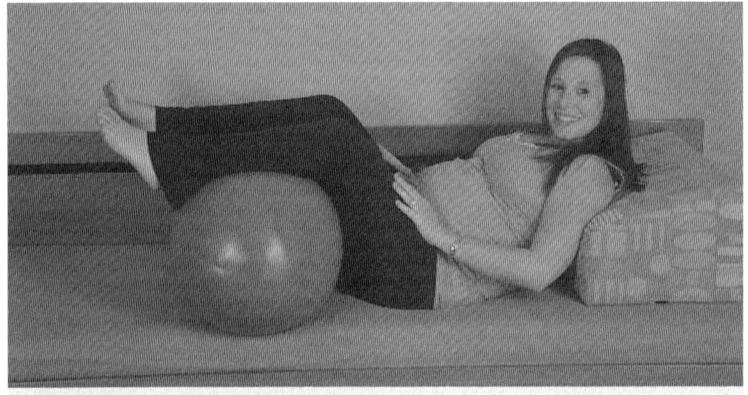

Photo © Premier Birth Tools LLC

> *I love the peanut ball and advise all my clients to get one for birth.*
>
> Yuen Kwan Chan, midwife, New York

I was working as an OB Tech in Mother Baby; one of the nurses asked me for assistance with her patient (she knew I was a doula and had peanut balls). She told me her patient was at 5 cm for three hours and was not progressing. I asked about the patient and if she had an epidural and other information. I introduced myself, told my story, and explained the peanut ball. I assisted my nurse and we moved the patient to different positions, using the peanut ball. About three hours later she was complete and one hour later she delivered a beautiful baby boy without a Cesarean section. We all had a great time. The nurse and patient thanked me.

Paul Cobb, retired doula and Peanut Ball Ambassador, Ohio

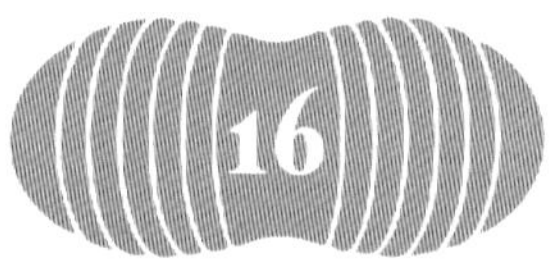

THE FUTURE OF PEANUT BALL

"I was with a home birth client, who historically moves very slowly through her births. We used the peanut ball (after a long active phase) and she moved to pushing within an hour."

—Kyndal May, doula and Peanut Ball Ambassador, Idaho

NEW INFORMATION AND RESEARCH on peanut balls is created all the time, and it's exciting how far we have come in learning about this useful birth tool. As we move into the future, I have three goals:

1) MAKE PEANUT BALLS AVAILABLE IN EVERY COUNTRY TO DECREASE THE CESAREAN RATE

Only a few countries currently use peanut balls. We know that peanut balls are used in the United States, Canada, Mexico, Australia, the UK, China, India, Japan, Dominican Republic, United Arab Emirates, Germany, Indonesia, Netherlands, New Zealand, Puerto Rico, Spain, and several others. The United States is currently leading the way with the highest number of peanut balls in most hospitals, and I would love to see peanut balls in every hospital in the United States.

2) TRAIN ANYONE INVOLVED WITH BIRTH HOW TO CORRECTLY SIZE AND USE THE PEANUT BALL WITH THEIR CLIENTS

Our In-Service Training for Peanut Balls and Authorized Peanut Ball Trainers are helping us work toward this goal.

3) MORE RESEARCH WITH LARGE STUDIES

We're seeing new research all the time, but I also challenge each of you to do your own research. Those who can facilitate peanut ball research studies, please do so. We need studies in every setting: hospital, birthing center, and home births. We need evidence-based research that drives evidence-based practice.

We have a lot of work to do, but every time we add peanut balls to a new hospital, we're helping reduce the Cesarean rate. I challenge you to educate your local community about peanut balls and encourage your hospitals, birth centers, and home birth midwives to bring them to your area. Our Peanut Ball Ambassadors are working to do this in their communities, and we always love adding more ambassadors to our team. If you would like to train others how to use the peanut ball correctly, you may be interested in our Authorized Peanut Ball Trainer program.

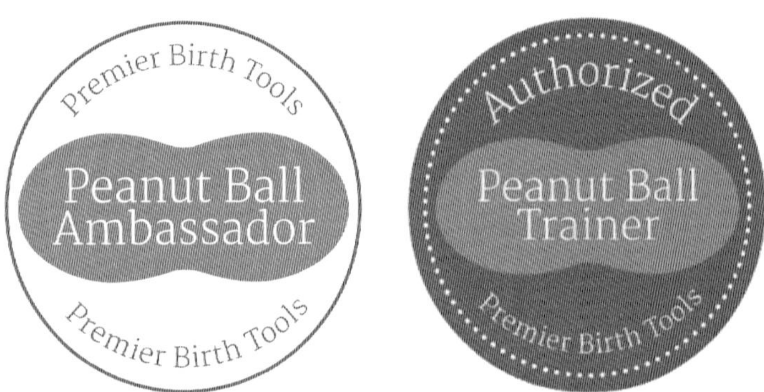

I have used the peanut ball for years in many birth settings including remote parts of the world! I love that it is a tool we can use when making diameter changes at all levels of the pelvis. It is highly effective for rotation and/or decent at the midpelvis especially when a person needs to stay in bed. The use of a peanut ball can help a labor to progress so other interventions are not needed!

Tammy Ryan, SpBT and Peanut Ball Ambassador, Iowa

PEANUT BALLS ARE REPORTEDLY USED IN THESE COUNTRIES

United Stated

- 13 Peanut Ball Trainers: premierbirthtools.com/authorized-peanut-ball-trainers/
- 60 Peanut Ball Ambassadors: premierbirthtools.com/peanut-ball-ambassadors/
- Every state has peanut balls, but not yet every hospital

Countries Outside the United States

Sixteen countries have reported using peanut balls (Ambassador application interviews, 2014–2021).

Australia

Heather Borradale, *Peanut Ball Ambassador, midwife*

"I work as a midwife at the Sunshine Coast Private Hospital and I donated two peanut balls—40 cm and 50 cm. I have since used them in labor several times, along with other midwifes in the unit. We know for sure that for two labors the patient was offered Cesarean sections or epidural-and-wait. Both women used a peanut ball and delivered vaginally. Apart from that, we have had about 11 births; three vacuum assisted and the rest vaginal. So everyone is very excited about it."

Jenna Cicchillitti, *Peanut Ball Ambassador, midwife*

"I love peanut balls. They are wonderful for labor and birth!"

Canada

Stephanie Assouline, *Authorized Peanut Ball Trainer*

"I love teaching nurses how to use the peanut ball correctly"

Adam Smith, *dad*

"The peanut ball is amazing and I saw it used at my wife's birth."

Jessica Wojtkowiak, *doula*

"Client's water broke with no contractions. After five hours, [the] baby was still high. [I] suggested that the client lay down and get some sleep, [and]placed the peanut ball between her legs. One hour later, [the] baby had moved down and into optimal position, and contractions where now five minutes apart. We had a baby. Love the peanut ball!"

Heather Crossan, *doula and childbirth educator trainer*

"Canadians need to have better access [to] this amazing tool and amazing info! I have been in talks with my local hospitals to donate peanut balls and provide training. I'm *so* excited to learn that this program exists, so I don't have to reinvent the wheel!"

Dominican Republic

Sary Mendez, *doula*

"I love the peanut balls! "

Germany

Verena Möllenkamp, *doula*

"I haven't been using the peanut ball at my own births, because at that time they were not available in my area. I have tried to use the peanut ball at one of my first birth attendances, but the midwifes did not accept the new tool. Now midwives are using the peanut ball more after they have seen how well it works."

India

Pratibha Kamath, *Peanut Ball Ambassador, nurse at Manipal College of*

Nursing, MAHE, manipal near Tiger Circle, Madhav Nagar Manipal, Karnataka, India

"I am excited to teach about peanut balls to nurses in India!"

Indonesia

Dela Jaskara, *childbirth educator*

"I love the peanut ball!"

Japan

Amanda Dodson, *Peanut Ball Ambassador*

"Peanut Balls are an amazing tool to use in labor and birth!"

Netherlands

Marloes Faber, *midwife, Peanut Ball Amabassador, The Netherlands*

"In the birth center with a home-midwife, a nulliparous stall at 5 cm dilated, high caput. Then tried their familiar positions and empty her bladder. Then they wanted to refer her to the medical ward for oxytocin IV. The doula/nurse there, who was informed about the peanut ball through me, suggested the peanut ball and explained. The midwife and the woman in labor agreed. Fifty-five minutes later, there was progression and she had a beautiful natural birth at the birth center without medical interventions!"

New Zealand

Elizabeth Good, *midwife*

"I am excited to disseminate this peanut ball information here in New Zealand. I have three hospitals and the New Zealand College of midwives interested we now have peanut balls! "

Puerto Rico

Estefanía Diez Gradín, *nurse*

"Peanut balls are amazing for labor!"

Ambar Rivera, *doula and childbirth educator from Puerto Rico*

"Puerto Rico has one if not the highest Cesarean rates, worldwide, and also the highest of the United States. I'm personally very committed to changing that, even if done one birth at a time. Using the peanut ball will help!"

Spain

Katherine Suarez Mix, *nurse from Alicante, La Nucia, Spain*

"I am excited about using peanut balls in Spain."

United Arab Emirates Dhabi

Mayte Miguel, *doula*

"I am a UK trained midwife. I now live in Abu Dhabi where birth is very medicalized with high rates of epidural and Cesarean section. I feel the community would benefit immensely from the use of the peanut ball. I would like to bring it to our doula community. Sadly, not many of the doulas here have heard about it or know how to use it to its full potential. I am excited about educating our birth professionals—midwives, doulas, educators—on the use and benefits of the peanut ball."

United Kingdom

Emma Trollope, *Peanut Ball Ambassador, midwife*

"I used a peanut ball for a primigravida being induced in labor with an epidural. By the end of my 12-hour shift, she progressed from 2 cm dilated, 50 percent effaced, high head, to fully dilated and presenting part had descended well. We changed position[s] regularly, using the peanut ball, which not only helped with the descent of the presenting part, but also with reducing any risk of pressure sores and dilation."

FUNDRAISERS

Help get peanut balls in every Labor and Delivery unit in the United States and the world. Fundraise and donate a peanut ball to every hospital, birthing center, and home-birth midwife. This will assist us in our goal to have a peanut ball in every birthing facility in the world.

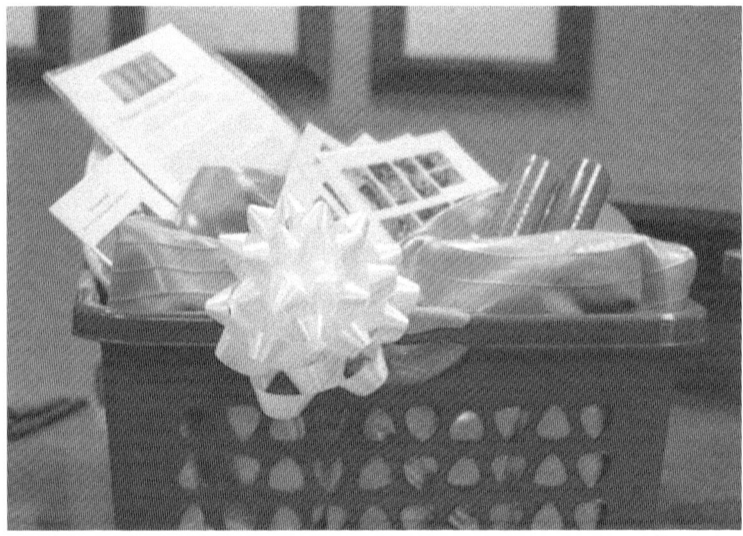

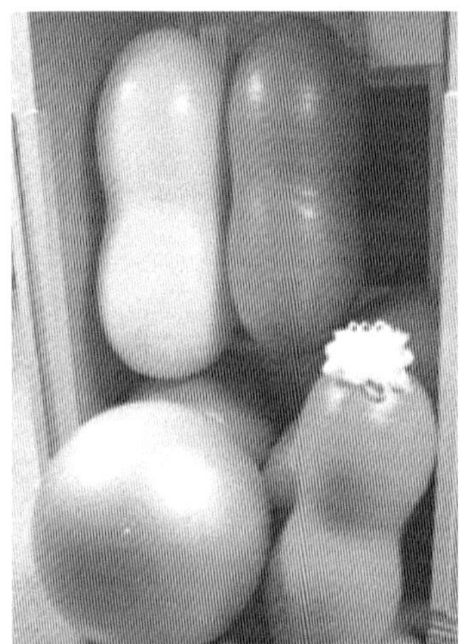

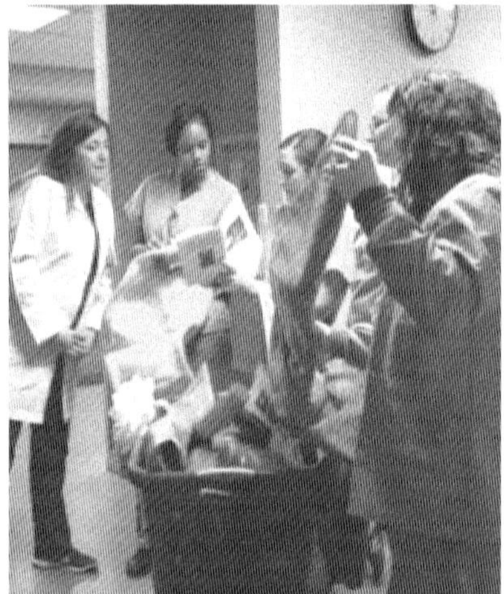

A successful fundraiser to purchase peanut balls for Gateway Medical Center in Clarksville, Tennessee, April 2016.

Photo courttesy of Heidi Duncan, CBD (CBI), Expecting New Life

I want for all of my perinatal nurses to have the tools and knowledge available to minimize the need for Cesarean Delivery, unless medically indicated.

Cheryl Fortenberry, nurse, Texas

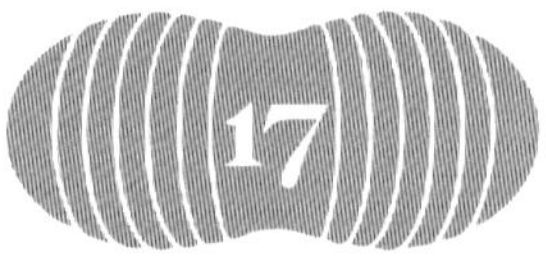

CONCLUSION

"Peanut Balls are an amazing essential tool that should be available at every birth."

—Cheri Grant, nurse, Oklahoma

THE PEANUT BALL IS AN essential tool that should be in every hospital Labor and Delivery unit, birthing center, home birth, and doula bag. It is a low-tech tool that has significantly changed the length of labor in first and second stages. The peanut ball is especially efficient when used with a client who has an epidural and is unable to move in bed to rotate the baby to a more optimal fetal position. It is perfect for helping clients to change positions in labor and feel supported, while enhancing the process of labor and birth. Peanut balls are an indispensable tool in today's maternity care that do not need a doctor's order.

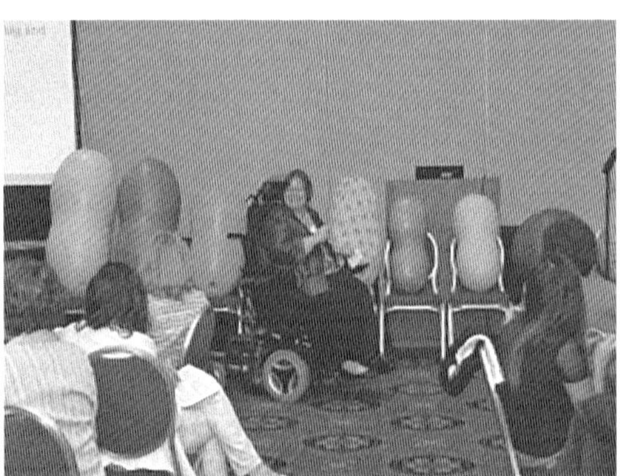

"The Peanut Ball Lady" Cheri Grant RN, ICCE, CLC, ICBD, CLD, CD BDT (DONA).

APPENDICES

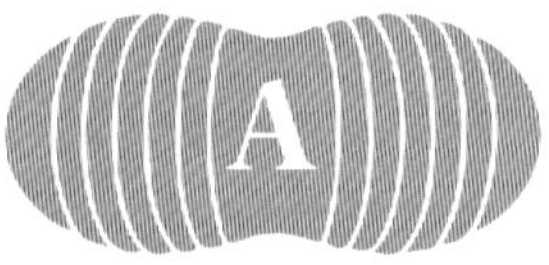

EVIDENCE-BASED RESEARCH ARTICLES

"We have used peanuts balls (and birth balls) since I have been at my current hospital. After taking the Spinning Babies® training, I have used them a lot more and have encouraged/shown other nurses, parents, and patients' different positions to be in, based on where they are in labor."

—Tracy Claxton, nurse, Colorado

MORE RESEARCH AND larger studies are needed, but there is current evidence-based research that can be shared.

SIGNIFICANT FINDINGS IN PEANUT BALL STUDIES

Hickey, L., Savage, J. (2019) Effect of Peanut Ball and Position Changes in Women Laboring with an Epidural. NFWH: Nursing for Women's Health WHONN June 2019 , Volume 23, Issue 3, Pages 245–252 DOI: https://doi.org/10.1016/j.nwh.2019.04.004

Quick Details

- **Overall, women in the peanut ball group were 50 percent less likely to have a Cesarean birth**
- Women who had dilated up to 4 cm or less were 61 percent less likely to have a Cesarean birth

Jena Palladino, Jena, Severi, Erica R., Bowman, Donna, Nurse-Driven Labor Initiatives to Reduce Cesarean Rates Journal of Obstetric, Gynecologic & Neonatal Nursing JOGNN June 2019 Volume 48, Issue 3, Supplement, Pages S28–S29 DOI: https://doi.org/10.1016/j.jogn.2019.04.048

Quick Details (MOST EFFECTIVE)

- Each nurse had to attend a hands-on, in-service training and skills lab competency checklist before the study began
- **Six months after the training, the researchers saw a 6 percent decrease in the Cesarean rate**
- Their research shows nurses need to be properly trained on peanut balls for them to be most effective

Tussey, C. & Botsios, E. (2011). Decrease the length of labor with the use of a labor ball with patients that receive an epidural. Journal of Obstetric, Gynecological, & Neonatal Nursing, vol 40(Supplement s1), S105-S106. DOI: 10.1111/j.1552-6909.2011.01243_25.x

Quick Details

- Decreases 1st Stage by 90 minutes
- Decreases 2nd stage by 23 min
- **Decreases Cesarean rate by 13 percent**

As a nurse, I have advocated for peanut balls to be used on my unit since I became a Labor and Delivery nurse. I moved from being a doula into nursing, and brought my "bag of tricks" with me. My coworkers really love the peanut ball!

Alicia Hicks, nurse, Ohio

RESEARCH ARTICLES ON THE PEANUT BALL

Hickey, L., Savage, J. (2019) Effect of Peanut Ball and Position Changes in Women Laboring with an Epidural. NFWH: Nursing For Women's Health AWHONN June 2019 Volume 23, Issue 3, Pages 245–252 DOI: https://doi.org/10.1016/j.nwh.2019.04.004 Effect of Peanut Ball and Position Changes in Women Laboring With an Epidural - Nursing for Women's Health (nwhjournal.org)

Logan, L, Stettler, S. (2019) "Reduction of Primary Cesarean Birth Rate in a Rural Hospital Driven By Nurse-Initiated Peanut Ball Use in Active Labor" JOGNN: Journal of Obstetric, Gynecologic & Neonatal Nursing June 2019 Volume 48, Issue 3, Supplement, Page S110 Reduction of Primary Cesarean Birth Rate in a Rural Hospital Driven By Nurse-Initiated Peanut Ball Use in Active Labor - Journal of Obstetric, Gynecologic & Neonatal Nursing (jognn.org)

Mercier, R.J. & Kwan. M. (2018). Impact of Peanut ball device on the duration of active labor: A randomized control trial. American Journal of Perinatology, 2018 March 6. doi: 10.1055/s-0038-1636531. Thieme E-Journals - American Journal of Perinatology / Abstract (thieme-connect.de)

Roth, C., Dent, S., Parfitt, S. E., Hering, S. & Bay, R. (2016). Randomized controlled trial of use of the peanut ball during labor. MCN: The Journal of Maternal Child Nursing. 41(3), 140-146. ISSN: 0361-929X doi: 10.1097/NMC.0000000000000232 Randomized Controlled Trial of Use of the Peanut Ball During... : MCN: The American Journal of Maternal/Child Nursing (lww.com)

Palladino, Jena, Severi, Erica R., Bowman, Donna, "Nurse-Driven Labor Initiatives to Reduce Cesarean Rates" Journal of Obstetric, Gynecologic & Neonatal Nursing JOGNN June 2019 Volume 48, Issue 3, Supplement, Pages S28–S29 DOI: https://doi.org/10.1016/j.jogn.2019.04.048 Nurse-Driven Labor Initiatives to Reduce Cesarean Rates - Journal of Obstetric, Gynecologic & Neonatal Nursing (jognn.org)

Tussey, C. M., Botsios, E., Gerkin, R. D., Kelly, L. A., Gamez, J., & Mensik, J. (2015). Reducing Length of Labor and Cesarean Surgery Rate Using a Peanut Ball for Women Laboring With an Epidural. The Journal of Perinatal Education, 24(1), 16-24. doi:10.1891/1058-1243.24.1.16 Reducing Length of Labor and Cesarean Surgery Rate Using a Peanut Ball for Women Laboring With an Epidural | Springer Publishing

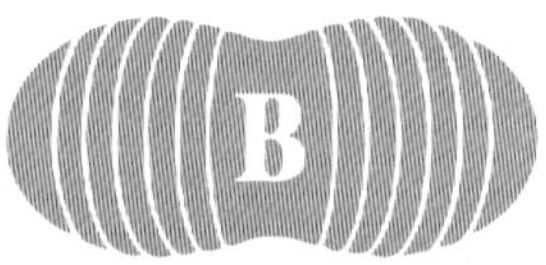

ARTICLES ON PEANUT BALLS

"As a nurse, I have used a peanut ball with pretty much all my patients, especially at night when they have an epidural and just want to sleep. I use it and turn them throughout the shift and their cervixes change! Even when everyone else is so skeptical!"

—Carolyn Nelson, nurse, Maryland

BELOW ARE THE LATEST articles as of publishing, updated lists can be found on the Premier Birth Tools research page.

Ahmadpour, Parivash, Mohammad-Alizadeh-Charandabi, Sakinah, Doosti, Rana, Mirghafourvand, Mojgan *Use of the peanut ball during labour: A systematic review and meta-analysis* Nurs Open. 2021 Mar 27. doi: 10.1002/nop2.844. Use of the peanut ball during labour: A systematic review and meta-analysis - PubMed (nih.gov)

Bell, Amy D. & Joy, Saju & Gullo, Susan, More. (2017). Implementing a Systematic Approach to Reduce Cesarean Birth Rates in Nulliparous Women. Journal of Obstetrics, Gynecology, American College of Obstetricians and Gynecologists (ACOG), 130(5):1082-1089. Implementing a Systematic Approach to Reduce Cesarean Birth... : Obstetrics & Gynecology (lww.com)

Ezuma, Ndidiamaka (2020) The Use of the Peanut Ball on Nulliparous Women Laboring With An Epidural Directed Scholarly Project complete_311220083154.pdf (doctorsofnursingpractice.org)

Grenvik JM, Rosenthal E, Saccone G, Della Corte L, Quist-Nelson J, Gerkin RD, Gimovsky AC, Kwan M, Mercier R, Berghella V. Peanut ball for decreasing length of labor: A systematic review and meta-analysis of randomized controlled trials. Eur J Obstet Gynecol Reprod Biol. 2019 Nov;242:159–165. doi: 10.1016/j.ejogrb.2019.09.018. Epub 2019 Sep 20 Peanut ball for decreasing length of labor: A systematic review and meta-analysis of randomized controlled trials - PubMed (nih.gov)

Clutter, L. B. & Grant, C. B. (2015). Peanut Balls: Improving Options for Women Laboring with an Epidural. Australian Midwifery News, 15(3). 36–37. Australian-College-of-Midwives-Pages-36-37-from-AMN-Spring-2015-peanut-ball-article-FINAL-HiRes.pdf (premierbirthtools.com)

Craig, B., Grant, C. B., & Rice, A. (2014). Length of labor reduced through use of peanut ball: A retrospective study. Unpublished manuscript.

Clutter, L. B. & Grant, C. B. (2014). The peanut ball: A remarkable labor support tool. International Doula, 22(4), 12–15. Peanut-

BallArticleInternationalDoula2014.pdf (premierbirthtools.com)

Grant, C. (2021) Premier Birth Tools Peanut Ball Informational Nurse and Doula Packet. Peanut Ball Nurse Packet - Premier Birth Tools

Lee & Crawford (2018) Peanut Ball Use by Women Labor: A review of Literature http://kpscnursingresearch.org/wp- admin/images/Forms/Literative%20Evidence%20Summaries/Peanut%20 Ball%20Literature%20Review_FINAL_April%202018.pdf Peanut Ball Literature Review_FINAL_April 2018.pdf (kpscnursingresearch.org)

Lythgoe, A. (2014). Peanut balls for labor—A valuable tool for promoting progress? A Research Blog About Healthy Pregnancy, Birth & Beyond. Lamaze International. Retrieved from http:// www.scienceandsensibility.org/?p=8166 Peanut Balls for Labor - A Valuable Tool for Promoting Progress? (lamaze.org)

Outland, L., & Alvarado, Y. (2020). Preventing cesareans with peanut ball use. Journal of Nursing Education and Practice, 10(1).https://www.researchgate.net/profile/Lauren_Outland/ publication/336728971_Preventing_cesareans_with_peanut_ball_use/links/5dfae0364585159aa487e60b/Preventing cesareans-with-peanut-ball-use.pdf Preventing-cesareans-with-peanut-ball-use.pdf (researchgate.net)

Simkin, P. Hanson, L. & Ancheta, R. (2017). The Labor Progress Handbook (4nd ed.) Malden, MA: Blackwell Science.

Smith H & Peterson N & Lagrew D & Main E. (2016) Toolkit to support vaginal birth and reduce primary cesareans: a quality improvement toolkit. Stanford (CA) Maternal Quality Care Collaborative CMQCC- Updated 2018 with peanut ball section (PDF) Toolkit to Support Vaginal Birth and Reduce Primary Cesareans A Quality Improvement Toolkit | Christian Orejudos - Academia.edu

Tully, G (2020) Changing Birth on Earth: A Midwife and nurse's guide to using physiology to avoid another unnecessary cesarean. Maternity House Publishing

GRADUATE THESIS, DISSERTATIONS, AND CAPSTONES ON THE PEANUT BALL

After completing my doctoral capstone project on the use of the peanut ball to reduce the Cesarean Delivery rate, I was even more convinced of the benefit of such a low-cost intervention. Increased use of the peanut ball allows for greater maneuverability of the maternal pelvis and potential reductions in the Cesarean section rate in many instances. Coupled with the increase in spontaneous vaginal deliveries and patient satisfaction, expected results could lead to a turnaround in the cost of a higher Cesarean rate—both financially and health-risk wise.

Dr. Jennifer Klump, DNP, CNM, RN, Illinois

Honaker, Megan Elizabeth, (2021) "The Use of a Peanut Ball During Labor in Nulliparous Term Singleton Vertex Pregnancies to Decrease the Primary Cesarean Rate: An Evidence-Based Practice Improvement Project" (2021). Graduate Publications and Other Selected Works - Doctor of Nursing Practice (DNP). https://trace.tennessee.edu/dnp/3 The Use of a Peanut Ball During Labor in Nulliparous Term Singleton Vertex Pregnancies to Decrease the Primary Cesarean Rate: An Evidence-Based Practice Improvement Project (tennessee.edu)

Klump, Jennifer S., (2017) "Use of the Peanut Ball to Reduce Cesarean Rate" (Publication No. 26) [Doctoral dissertation, University of Northern Colorado]. https://digscholarship.unco.edu/capstones/26 Use of the Peanut Ball to Reduce Cesarean Rate (unco.edu)

Payton, Carol L., (2015). Use of the Peanut Ball to Decrease First and Second Stages of Labor Graduate Theses, Dissertations, and Capstones, Paper 14. Retrieved from http://scholarworks.bellarmine.edu/cgi/viewcontent.cgi?article=1013&context=tdc Use of the Peanut Ball to Decrease First and Second Stages of Labor (premier-birthtools.com)

ADDITIONAL CITATIONS FOR THIS BOOK ON THE PEANUT BALL

Bueno-Lopez .V, Fuentelsaz-Gallego .C, Casellas-Caro .M, Falgueras-Serrano. M, Crespo-Berros .S, Silvano-Cocinero. A, Alcaine-Guisado . C, Fuentes .M, Carreras. E, Terré-Rull .C, (2018) " Efficiency of the modified Sims maternal position in the rotation of persistent occiput posterior position during labor: A randomized clinical trial Birth ." Birth Dec;45(4):385–392. doi: 10.1111/birt.12347. https://pubmed.ncbi.nlm.nih.gov/29537658/

Cockeram, Mindy (2020). Narrow the Knees to Push with Ease: Challenge The Norm and Get The Job Done! A Research Blog About Healthy Pregnancy, Birth & Beyond. Lamaze International. Retrieved from Narrow the Knees to Push with Ease: Challenge The Norm and Get The Job Done! (lamaze.org)

Heffernan, C. (2016). A brief history of the Swiss ball. Retrieved from https://physicalculturestudy.com/2017/12/27/a-brief-history-of-the-swiss-ball-2/

Opening the Bottom of the Pelvis for Pushing -Outlet Opening (2019, MamasteFit Training)

Perez, Polly (2000) Birth Balls: Use of Physical Therapy Balls in Maternity, Cutting Edge Press

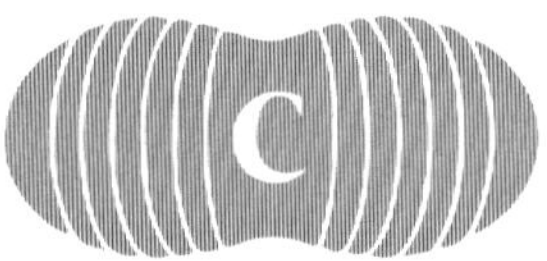

POSTER PRESENTATIONS ON PEANUT BALLS

"In Novemeber of 2017, a nurse manager wrote me, 'Traveling nurses have been asking why we do not have peanut balls. I guess it is time to order a peanutbBall starter kit.'"

—Antelope Valley Hospital, Lancaster, CA

BELOW ARE THE LATEST poster presentations, as of publishing. Visit Premier Birth Tools research page to see an updated list.

Alvarado, Yolanda, Outland, Lauren,,Menchaca, Angelica, Strong, Niki. (2017). Promoting the Progress of Labor with the Peanut Ball. Journal of Obstetric, Gynecologic & Neonatal Nursing, Volume 46 (Issue 3), Supplement, 23. Retrieved from http://www.jognn.org/article/S0884-2175(17)30127-2/abstract Promoting the Progress of Labor With the Peanut Ball - Journal of Obstetric, Gynecologic & Neonatal Nursing (jognn.org)

DeOliveira, E. (2016). EBP Poster Presentation: Can the use of peanut balls reduce the length of labor? Retrieved from https://www.youtube.com/watch?v= EBP Poster Presentation-Can the Use of Peanut Balls Reduce the Length of Labor? - YouTube

Bell, Catherine (2018) Effectiveness of Using the Peanut Ball to shorten the first and Second Stage of labor https://sigma.nursingrepository.org/bitstream/handle/10755/623757/Bell_Info_89909.pdf;sequence=2 Bell_Info_89909.pdf;sequence=2 (nursingrepository.org)

Bookwalter, Amy. (2016). Peanut Ball Positions. Pictorial Home Birth Poster Presentation at 2017 DONA International Convention

Clutter, L. B. (2016) The Peanut Ball: A useful Tool for Labor & Delivery Support 2016 Family Nursing International Conference The Peanut Ball: A Useful Tool for Labor and Delivery Support (hilarispublisher.com)

Evans, Sarah J, & Cremering, Michelle M. Use of Peanut Labor Ball for Pelvic Positioning for Nulliparous Women Following Epidural Anesthesia. Journal of Obstetric, Gynecologic, & Neonatal Nursing, (2016) Volume 45, Issue 3, Page S47. Use of Peanut Labor Ball for Pelvic Positioning for Nulliparous Women Following Epidural Anesthesia - Journal of Obstetric, Gynecologic & Neonatal Nursing (jognn.org)

Martinez-Rodriguez. A, Stairhime, C, Use of Birthing Tools to Decrease Labor Times Houston Methodist Willowbrook https://www.texaschildrens.org/sites/default/files/uploads/documents/health_professionals/kaleidoscope/Day%202%20Birthing%20Tools.pdf

Potter, K. & Will, S. (2020) Increasing Use of the Peanut Ball in Labor JOGNN Volume 49, Issue 6, Supplement, S46, November 01, 2020 DOI: https://doi.org/10.1016/j.jogn.2020.09.079 Increasing Use of the Peanut Ball in Labor - Journal of Obstetric, Gynecologic & Neonatal Nursing (jognn.org)

Schmidt, M. & Roach, A. (2015). A peanut and a pelvis: A simple change to facilitate labor and delivery. Science Internship Program: Nursing Care at Cleveland Clinic. Retrieved from: http://civiceducation.clevelandclinic.org/getattachment/7cad7959-f19c-4f7b-b5a4-b7a4259ad476/A-Peanut-and-a-Pelvis-A-Simple-Change-to-Facilitat.aspx Slide 1 (clevelandclinic.org)

Tussey, C. & Botsios, E. (2011). Decrease the length of labor with the use of a labor ball with patients that receive an epidural. Journal of Obstetric, Gynecological, & Neonatal Nursing, 40(Supplement s1), S105-S106. DOI: 10.1111/j.1552-6909.2011.01243_25.x Use of a Labor Ball to Decrease the Length of Labor in Patients Who Receive an Epidural - Tussey - 2011 - Journal of Obstetric, Gynecologic, & Neonatal Nursing - Wiley Online Library

> *If we can prevent even one Cesarean section, we feel this was successful! We love the peanut ball!*
>
> **Katie Wiederholt, nurse at Mercy Medical Center, Dubuque, Iowa**

"At our facility, we completed a retrospective analysis of six months of data for use with and without the peanut ball for positioning after epidural placement in the nulliparous, term, singleton, vertex patient population (NTSV).

- The study included 108 pre-peanut ball intervention subjects and 105 post-peanut ball intervention subjects
- Staff were educated on the use of the peanut ball at a staff meeting with an instructional video and demonstration
- Instructional posters were placed in the Labor and Delivery break-room and each labor room for reference and patient education
- Peanut balls were used on selected patients after placement of epidural versus standard positioning with pillows
- Size of ball was selected based on patient's height
- Patient repositioning was done according to policy
- Hourly during the first stage of labor
- Every 15–30 minutes during the second stage of labor

Overall there was an 8.8 percent decrease in the Cesarean section rate of the post-intervention group. Despite the fact there were more diabetic patients, larger babies, and more inductions of labor, which all increase the risk of a Cesarean Delivery.

Changes in practice, to using the peanut ball ,have been well-received by patients, nurses ,and physicians."

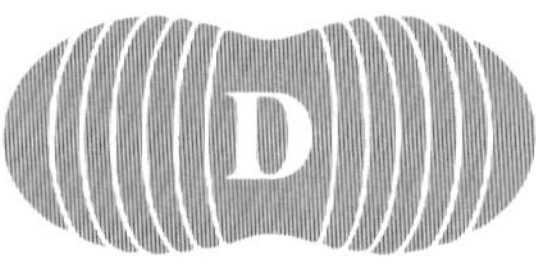

CLINICAL TRIALS ON PEANUT BALLS

"A study was being done at the hospital in Evansville, Indiana, to see if it decreased the Cesarean section rate. It was great to be a part of this and—yes—it did work."

—Cheryl Yow, nurse, Massachusetts

BELOW ARE THE LATEST clinical trials as of publishing. Visit Premier Birth Tools research page to see an updated list.

Beyazıt, Ankara Yildirim University2 March (2021) The Effect of Using a Birthing Ball (Peanut Ball) During Labor on the Labor Process https://trialbulletin.com/lib/entry/ct-04729426

Birthing Ball (Peanut Ball) Positions: Labor Pain Clinical Trial... (trialbulletin.com)

D'Angelo, R. & Harris, L. (2016). Do peanut shaped birthing balls reduce the length of labor in patients with epidural analgesia? ClinicalTrials.gov Identifier: NCT02539563. Retrieved from https://clinicaltrials.gov/ct2/show/NCT02539563?term=Peanut+Ball&rank=1 Do Peanut Shaped Birthing Balls Reduce the Length of Labor in Patients With Epidural Analgesia? - Full Text View - ClinicalTrials.gov

Mackeen, Awathif D, Quinn. Shantel T (2019) Geisinger Medical Center Reducing Cesarean Delivery Rate in Obese Patients Using the Peanut Ball https://clinicaltrials.gov/ct2/show/NCT03772886 Reducing Cesarean Delivery Rate in Obese Patients Using the Peanut Ball - Full Text View - ClinicalTrials.gov

Milton, Sarah H (2020) Using the Peanut Exercise Ball to Reduce Cesarean Section Rates: A Randomized Controlled Trial https://clinicaltrials.gov/ct2/show/NCT02899260 Using the Peanut Exercise Ball to Reduce Cesarean Section Rates: A Randomized Controlled Trial - Full Text View - ClinicalTrials.gov

Stulz, V., Campbell, D., Yin, B. et al. Pilot Feasibility Stud (2018) 4: 156. https://doi.org/10.1186/s40814-018-0346-9 using a peanut ball during labor versus not using a peanut ball during labor for women using an epidural: study protocol for a randomized controlled pilot study https://pilotfeasibilitystudies.biomedcentral.com/track/pdf/10.1186/s40814-018-0346-9 Using a peanut ball during labour versus not using a peanut ball during labour for women using an epidural: study protocol for a randomised controlled pilot study (biomedcentral.com)

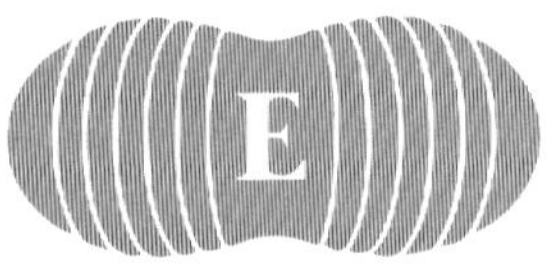

PODCASTS ON PEANUT BALLS

"I was on my way to my client's birth two hours away, and we had previously discussed using the peanut ball when she received an epidural. On my long drive I was listening to the evidence-based births podcast, on peanut ball use, to prepare for her birth to make sure I knew what I was doing. Sure enough, the baby bullet worked! After rolling her back and forth every 30 minutes or so, she had her baby two hours later. Super-fast pushing phase!"

—Janelle Trichell, doula, Louisiana

EVIDENCE BASED BIRTH PODCAST

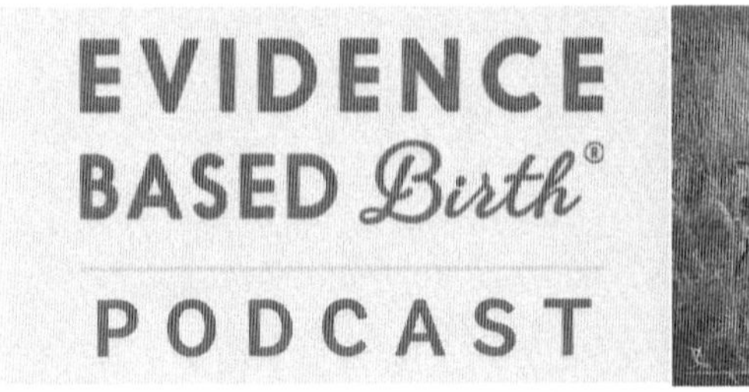

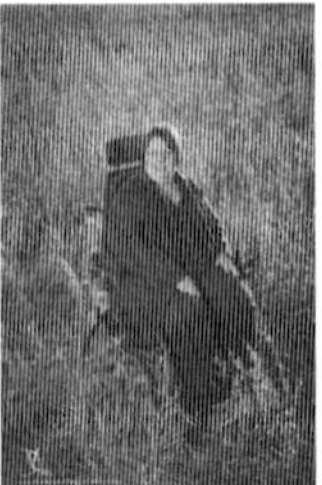

EBB45 - How do Peanut Balls Support Labor?
Cheri Grant RN-The Peanut Ball Lady

Evidence Based Birth EBB 45 - How do Peanut Balls Support Labor? With Cheri Grant, September 26, 2018 EBB 45 - How do peanut balls support labor? - Evidence Based Birth®

"A lot of nurses and doulas and midwives just think that the only way you can use a peanut ball is by placing the patient on their side and putting the peanut ball between their legs. And that's not always the correct position for the patient, for their stage of labor."

—Cheri Grant, RN, podcast interview with Evidence Based Birth®

"Peanut balls currently are an extremely popular invention. It's non-medical; they do contribute to labor support and maximizing fetal descent. They do contribute to decreased maternal pain. Peanut balls are cost effective and they really don't have any untoward side effects."

—Cheri Grant, RN, podcast interview with Evidence Based Birth®

In this week's podcast I interview Cheri Grant RN, ICCE, CLC, IBCD, CLD, CD BDT(DONA), known in the birth world as "The Peanut Ball Lady." She is the founder, chief contributor, and inspiration for Premier Birth Tools. For over 42 years, she has served women as a Labor and Delivery nurse, childbirth educator, lactation consultant, national speaker, author, doula, and doula trainer. She has helped with well over 2,700 deliveries in the span of her career. Cheri is also the founder of Tulsa Doulas, a community group that has helped train and support doulas for over 20 years. Cheri's interest in peanut balls began when she first saw their use in labor in 1985. At that time, they were just straddled. In the 2000s, the usage of peanut balls was refined to the Side-Lying Position, and interest in them began to grow among birth professionals. They are used with and without an epidural, and can be effective in shortening labor. Premier Birth Tools promotes education via its website, as well as Peanut Ball Ambassadors and Authorized Peanut Ball Trainers. Cheri discusses peanut ball positions and other new information on this tool.

> *I learned more about peanut balls after listening to Cheri Grant's Podcast on Evidence Based Birth. I am excited about using peanut ball here in Spain.*
>
> Katherine Suarez Mix, nurse, Alicante, La Nucia, Spain

YOGA | BIRTH | BABIES PODCAST

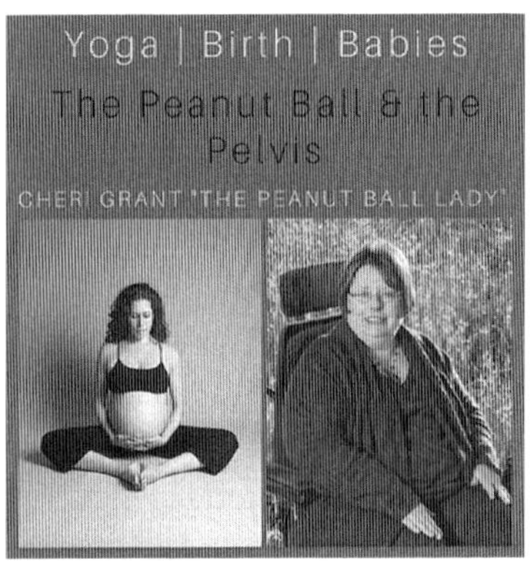

Yoga Birth Babies – The Peanut Ball and the Pelvis with Cheri Grant, RN, the "Peanut Ball Lady" September 16, 2019.

Prenatal Yoga Center | The Peanut Ball and the Pelvis with Cheri Grant the "Peanut Ball Lady".

In this episode of Yoga | Birth | Babies, I speak with Cheri Grant, also known worldwide as the "Peanut Ball Lady". Cheri explains how peanut balls are incorporated into labor and how they can positively effect labor. She goes into detail about how the different positions of a peanut ball can open the pelvis to help with fetal positioning, leading to a more functional birth. For pregnant people and birth workers, this conversation is a must!

In this episode:

- Learn about Cheri and how she got into birth work
- How Cheri got the nickname "Peanut Ball Lady"
- What is a peanut ball?
- Why peanut balls are helpful tool for labor

- All about peanut balls and the pelvis
- Data supporting the use of a peanut ball for a shortened labor
- How peanut balls can help decrease Cesarean births
- How peanut balls help with fetal position during labor
- Recommendations for how peanut balls are to be used
- Reasons why someone would be advised *not* to use a peanut ball
- Finding the right size peanut ball for you
- How to best introduce the idea and involvement of a peanut ball if a care provider or hospital is not accustomed to birthing people using them
- One tip/piece of advice Cheri has for new and expectant parents

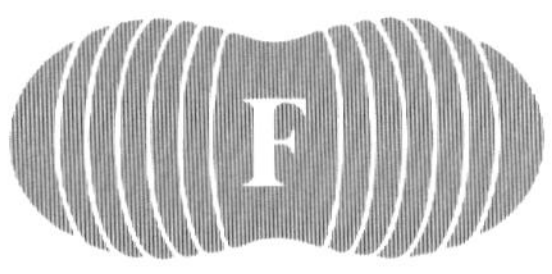

UNPUBLISHED RESEARCH ON PEANUT BALLS

"As a Labor and Delivery nurse, I feel strongly that the peanut ball was my most frequently used intervention after my patients received an epidural. They were happily accepted by patients. One of my patients, I remember vividly how she progressed from 5 cm to her baby being born in two hours as a first-time mom. For the first six hours of her labor, we had been trying different positions, movements and comforts. Then she requested an epidural at that point and was 5 cm. I settled her in a Side-Lying Position with the peanut ball, and rotated her side to side. Two hours later she welcomed her baby! I felt so happy for her to have reached the end of her birth story much quicker than we had imagined based on how slowly she had progressed from the beginning."

—Jerica Hortel, nurse, Arizona

THERE IS A SMALL amount of unpublished research on peanut balls that are retrospective studies. This was especially true when peanut balls were first introduced and talked about nationally in 2011.

The peanut ball was originally used in physical therapy. It has been used in labor support only recently. Tussey and Botsios (2011) reported their randomized, controlled trial on the use of the peanut ball (N=200: 107 with and 93 without peanut ball) with dramatic results. The primary outcome was a reduction of the first stage of labor by 90 minutes (p=0.006) and a decrease in the second stage by 22.3 minutes. The use of vacuum extraction and forceps were reduced in the group with the peanut ball. The study concluded that the use of the peanut ball, during labor for those with an epidural, significantly reduced the length of labor without adverse neonatal outcomes.

In an unpublished retrospective study in one Midwestern United States hospital (Grant, 2014) (N=218), use and non-use of the peanut ball was compared in samples of laboring women who received or did not receive an epidural. Of the patients with an epidural (N=174), 102 used a peanut ball 72 did not. In regards to time, the first stage was decreased by 102 minutes for those using the peanut ball, as compared with those who did not (with peanut ball- averaging 314.6 minutes versus without peanut ball averaging 211.9 minutes so difference of 102.1 minutes of the first stage). Comparing the Tussey and Botsios (2011) findings of a reduction by 90 minutes, this study revealed a comparable reduction of time

In the same unpublished retrospective study, the second stage of labor also demonstrated a reduction in time with use of the peanut ball. Of those with an epidural and no peanut ball, there was an average of 49.4 minutes and those with a peanut ball and an epidural had an average of 21.8 minutes during the second stage of labor. This demonstrates a reduction of 27.6 minutes for the second stage of labor. Comparing the Tussey and Botsios (2011) findings of a reduction by 22.3 minutes, this study again revealed a comparable reduction of time.

In the same unpublished retrospective study, (Grant, 2014) those without epidural were assessed. Out of the 218 total, 44 had no epidural. Of those, 28 used a peanut ball and 16 did not. Those who did not have an epidural and did not use the peanut ball had a first stage average of 326.4 minutes compared with a first stage time for those with the peanut ball of 217.9 minutes. This demonstrates a reduction of 108.5 minutes for the first stage of labor. Those who did not have an epidural and did not use the peanut ball had a second stage average of 41.8 minutes, compared with a second stage time for those with the peanut ball of 12.6 minutes. This demonstrates a reduction of 29.2 minutes for the first stage of labor.

In the level 1 hospital where this study was conducted, average Cesarean section rates were calculated for the year prior to the introduction of peanut ball use and the first year of its use. The rate decreased by 12 percent. While the reduction of rate can be attributed to various factors, the use of the peanut ball was a primary change in patient care. There was no significance difference for maternal age, gestational age of fetus, weight of newborn, augmentation of labor with oxytocin did not differ in any of the groups. No serious side effects or adverse reactions were ever noted when using the peanut ball. We need evidence-based research on the peanut ball.

Examples of using the peanut ball include:

- Epidural 6 cm Right 24 minutes then left 26 minutes (total 50 minutes) then complete +4 pushed 6 minutes
- **Time of Epidural and Peanut Ball to be Delivered (56 minutes)**
- Epidural 5 cm Right 20 minutes Left 21 minutes to complete +1 (total 41 minutes) pushed 28 minutes
- **Time of Epidural and Peanut Ball to be Delivered (1 hour 9 minutes)**
- Epidural 5 cm left 55 minutes to complete +2 (Total 55 minutes) pushed 20 minutes
- **Time of Epidural and Peanut Ball to be Delivered (1 hour 15 minutes)** All primips in above scenarios

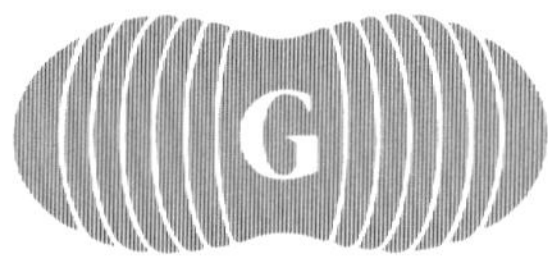

AUTHORIZED PEANUT BALL TRAINER VIDEOS

"Megan's peanut ball video was amazing! She explained how and when to put patients in specific positions—like external rotation and internal rotation—in relation to the patient's hips, not the baby's movements. . . . The part where she zooms in on her legs and feet to demonstrate fetal station and hip rotation was super beneficial."

—Kristen Miner, nurse and Peanut Ball Ambassador, Kansas

BELOW IS A COLLECTION of current peanut ball videos from our Authorized Peanut Ball Trainers. For an updated list of videos visit the Premier Birth Tools Resources page.

Assouline, Stephanie. (2017) Peanut Ball for labor. (Basic Advanced Positions) Authorized Peanut Ball Trainer Retrieved from https://www.youtube.com/watch?v=WcE-7wCNdTW0&t=145s

Duncan, Heidi. (2017). Peanut Ball Positions for Labor & Birth. Extensive and in-depth Peanut Ball Positions for Labor & Birth. Authorized Peanut Ball Trainer Retrieved from https://youtu.be/VlXOqs8q62g

Honaker, Megan. (2020) Using the Peanut Ball to Promote Vaginal Birth- What does a plié, windshield wipers and ruby red slippers have to do with a peanut ball? Authorized Peanut Ball https://youtu.be/kP_IeKkfDzU

Irby, Mandy (2017) Shorten labor faster with peanut ball. Nurse discussing internal and external rotation of hips using the peanut ball. Authorized Peanut Ball Trainer Retrieved from https://www.youtube.com/watch?v=B7mFvB9-HsU

Irby, Mandy (2019) What Does It Look Like to Push with Peanut Balls? // Peanut Balls in Labor - Nurse discussing pushing using the peanut ball Authorized Peanut Ball Trainer https://www.youtube.com/watch?v=28NXJfQ8w1Y

Scott, Marques. (2017). Labor with Peanut Balls. Nurse Fun, cute, and informational with basic and advance positions by a male Labor and Delivery nurse. Authorized Peanut Ball Trainer Retrieved from https://youtu.be/qxTfKlCXqUI

Turner, Heather. (2015) Four part video on how to size the peanut ball correctly for your client. Authorized Peanut Ball Trainer. Retrieved from https://www.youtube.com/playlist?list=PL5h-501qK0oo8FMy1UdWJZf_Dt9vqTIgAl

Whitlock, Emma. (2018) Peanut Ball Uses in Labor shows how to use peanut balls at home. Authorized Peanut Ball Trainer. Retrieved from https://www.youtube.com/watch?v=sOb2OJHGBwg

PEANUT BALL PUSHING POSITIONS VIDEOS

Cockeram , Mindy (2020). Narrow the Knees to Push with Ease: Challenge The Norm and Get The Job Done! A Research Blog About Healthy Pregnancy, Birth & Beyond. Lamaze International.Video in blog Retrieved from https://www.lamaze.org/Connecting-the-Dots/Post/narrow-the-knees-to-push-with-ease-challenge-the-norm-and160get-the-job-done-1

Irby, Mandy (2019) What Does It Look Like to Push with Peanut Balls? // Peanut Balls in Labor - Nurse discussing pushing using the peanut ball Authorized Peanut Ball Trainer https://www.youtube.com/watch?v=28NXJfQ8w1Y

MamasteFit Training (2019) This video does a great job of demonstrating opening the bottom of the pelvis for pushing outlet opening. https://www.youtube.com/watch?time_continue=1&v=sw8wR-2LRgo&feature=emb_logo Opening the Bottom of the Pelvis for Pushing -Outlet Opening

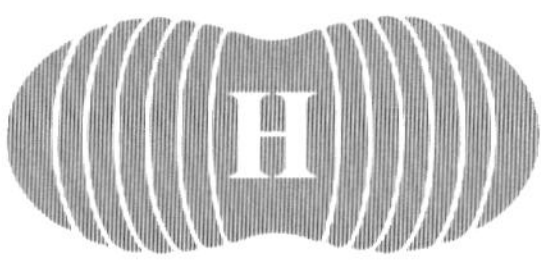

EDUCATIONAL TRAINING RESOURCES FOR PEANUT BALLS

"Premier Birth Tools provides excellent resources, inspiring educational presentations, and great products for every birthing person, childbirth educator, doula, and all birth providers. I love their products and include them in all my workshops and births."

—Debra Pascali-Bonaro, NJ of Orgasmic Birth: Doula Training, Childbirth Classes

WE'RE THRILLED TO OFFER several peanut ball educational materials and products at Premier Birth Tools. We've listed several of them here for your reference.

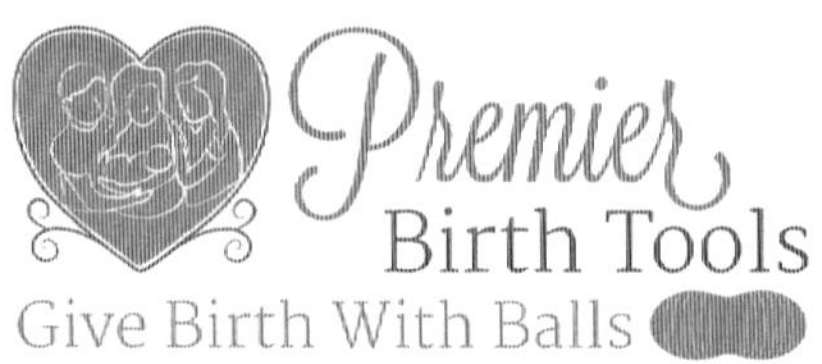

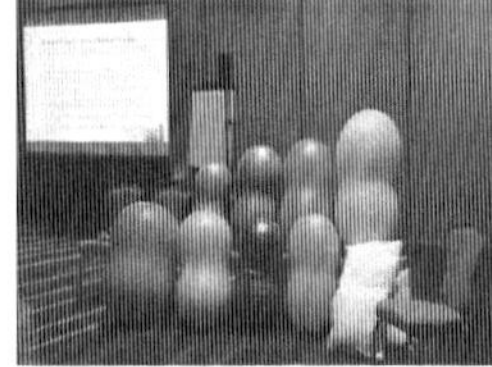
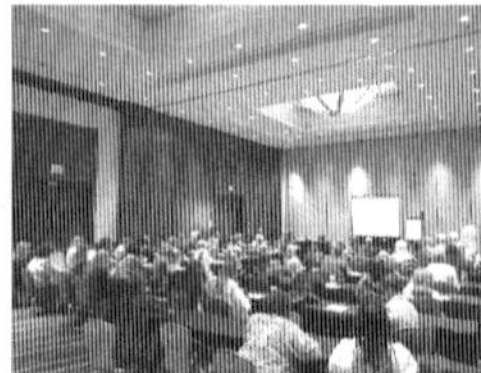
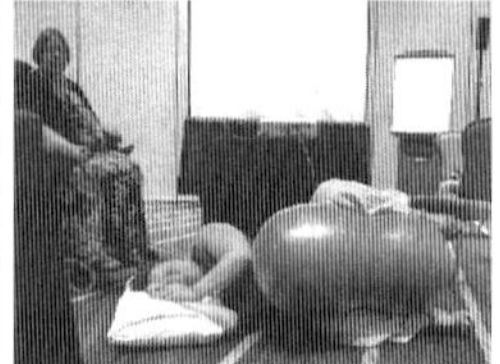

I took Cheri's session and was hooked on being able to help families and their nurses benefit from the use of the peanut ball. I use it in CBE class and now another hospital I teach at wants me to teach the nurses how to use it! Finally, it's catching on!

Kathy Shuman, childbirth educator, Michigan

Set of Five Peanut Ball Charts: Includes 50 peanut ball positions shown through 117 pictures. Orginal, new, pushing, internal, and external peanut ball positions from Premier Birth Tools

Peanut Ball Inservice Package to Train Nurses and Doulas: Peanut Ball In-Service Training Packages from Premier Birth Tools, includes peanut ball skills check list, a teaching outline, PowerPoint slides, set of five peanut ball charts, and more.

Tips for Nurses Using Peanut Balls: "How to Use the Peanut Ball" downloads from Premier Birth Tools

Peanut Ball PowerPoint: Peanut Ball Power Point from Premier Birth Tools

FREE Premier Birth Tools Peanut Ball Informational Packet: Peanut Ball Nurse Packet from Premier Birth Tools

Peanut Ball Videos: Peanut Ball videos from Premier Birth Tools

Set of 14 Childbirth Charts: Labor Charts with over 430 colorful pictures, showing 221 positions on an 8x10, two-sided chart. Childbirth Positions Charts – Set of Fourteen from Premier Birth Tools Perfect for nurses station or doula bag

Peanut Ball Training Information: premierbirthtools. We're always adding new tools to our website, so please check often for updates!

Peanut balls can be found on Premier Birth Tools, Amazon, Childbirth Graphics, and Aeromat websites. *If you are buying for a hospital, make sure peanut balls are hospital grade, which are thicker, hold up better, and are meant for multipurpose use.*

The peanut ball has been our Labor and Delivery nurse/midwife go-to for a stalled labor, especially with a patient who opted to have an epidural. Usually, we get the patient on her side with the peanut between her legs and soon she is feeling pressure, or sometimes an urge, to push. I am sad to find out we may be using them wrong at times. I see the benefit in the peanut ball, so I would love to learn more and help educate my community (multiple hospitals) about how to use them correctly. I am also adjunct faculty at the University of New Mexico and would love to share this information with our baby midwives—they might be able to teach other hospitals.

Nichele Salazar, CNM, midwife, New Mexico, heard Cheri speak at the Gold Midwifery Conference 2020

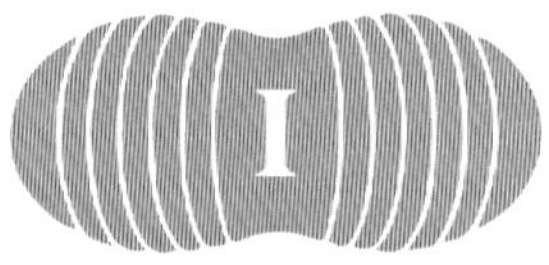

IN-SERVICE TRAINING FOR PEANUT BALLS

"Thank you so much! Your information is so helpful! I have increased my coworkers' knowledge and also our patients' knowledge. I have placed your charts in binders so the patients can browse through—whether they are having a natural delivery or a medicated delivery—to choose positions for labor."

—Amanda Hovey, labor and delivery nurse, Montana

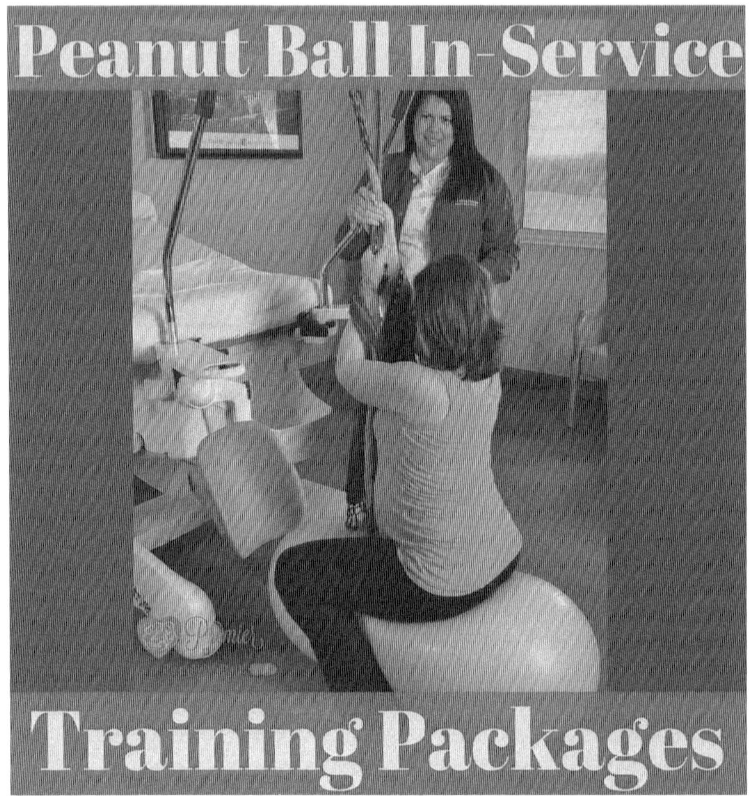

DOES YOUR STAFF KNOW how to correctly place the client's knees on the peanut ball if the baby is above the inlet, in the midpelvis, or in the outlet? Do they know internal and external rotation of the femur or thigh bones and which way they need to be in relation to the baby in the pelvis? Does your staff know all 50 basic and advanced peanut ball positions and when to use them? Does your staff know how to push with a peanut ball and all the peanut ball pushing positions? Does your staff know that one size peanut ball does not fit all clients, and how to correctly size a peanut ball? Does your staff know the contraindications for the peanut ball?

Many studies have found that staff value peanut ball education and would appreciate additional information (Potter, 2020) and (Honaker, 2021).

It is important to me that anyone who is training nurses, midwives, birth assistants, or doulas to use the peanut ball, is sharing the correct information. This is why we created our In-Service Training for Peanut Balls. The In-Service Training Package for Peanut Balls includes:

- **Set of 5 Peanut Ball Positions Charts** with over 182 pictures of 50 positions for the birthing bed
- **External and Internal Rotation Chart**, which determines the external and internal rotation of the femurs using the peanut ball. Chart features 19 pictures of 10 positions for the birthing bed
- **Evidence-Based Research** on the peanut ball
- **Peanut Ball Nurse Packet** to help nurses train and use the peanut ball correctly
- **Handout 1:** Proficiency Check-off List
- **Handout 2:** Tips for Nurses on How to Use the Peanut Ball
- **How to size the Peanut Balls** correctly
- **Peanut Ball PowerPoint** with PowerPoint slides, including all the research on peanut balls
- **Peanut Ball Booklet**
- **Peanut Ball Video** links by Authorized Peanut Ball Trainers (sent via email)
- **Basic and Advanced Peanut Ball Handout** with post-test

You can find out more about this training package by visiting our website: premierbirthtools.com

Important

MOST EFFECTIVE: Each nurse should attend a hands-on, in-service training and skills lab competency checklist.

A study done on peanut balls showed that there was a 6 percent decrease in the Cesarean rate after nurses were trained on peanut ball use after only six months (Palladino, 2019). It is so important to be sharing the correct information, and Premier Birth Tools and Authorized Peanut Ball Trainers makes that easy!

To properly train nurses for skills labs and in-services, we recommend purchasing Premier Birth Tools Peanut Ball In-service Training Package. It covers everything and includes several handouts, outlines, objectives, evidence-based research, proficiency skills checklist, test, updated PowerPoint, charts, and tips for nurses that are not covered in this book.

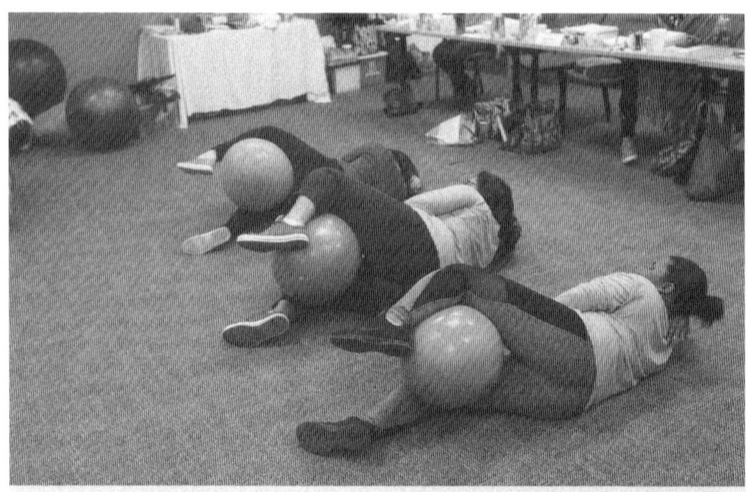

Peanut Ball Inservice Training: Learning how to correctly size a patient.
Photo © Premier Birth Tools LLC

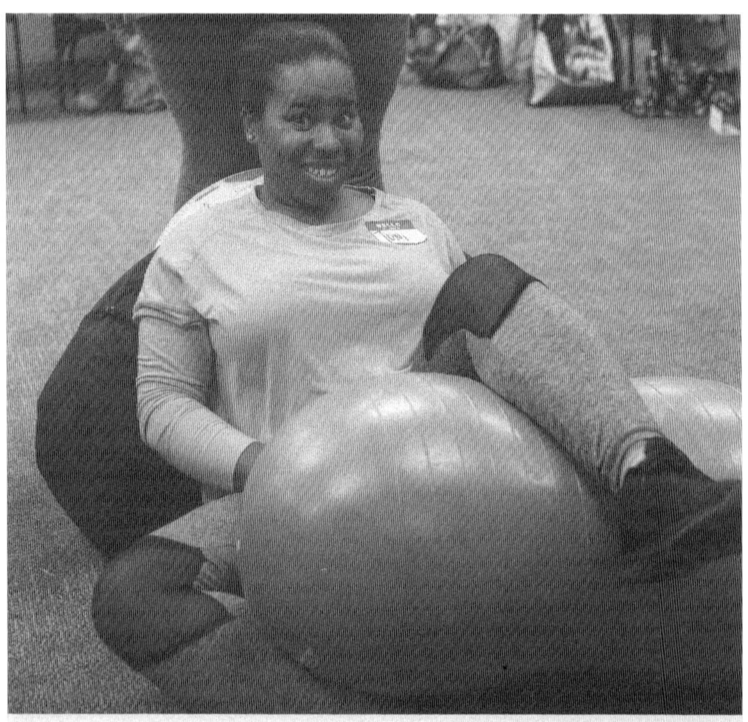

Peanut Ball Inservice Training: Return demonstration.
Photo © Premier Birth Tools LLC

NURSE SKILLS LABS AND IN-SERVICES SAMPLE

- Set up a skills lab
- Teach material provided in a new and updated Peanut Ball PowerPoint
- Distribute handouts, outline, objectives, evidence-based research, tips for nurses using peanut balls and have each nurse complete the test
- Have each nurse demonstrate, on each other, peanut ball positions on the charts
- Have nurse demonstrate how to properly size the peanut ball for their patient, noting there are four different sizes of peanut balls
- Have nurse demonstrate the different size of peanut ball in each of the different positions. (i.e., the Tuck Position takes a large size peanut ball, and the Semi-Sitting Lunge takes a smaller size peanut ball for each patient.)
- Perform sizing two different people on the correct size peanut ball in different positions.
- Have nurses verbally explain how to cover, clean, and store the peanut balls
- Show videos on how to use the peanut ball. *See Appendix G on videos*
- *Show all 5 Peanut Ball Charts with over 50 positions, using Peanut Ball.* These charts are included in the Peanut Ball In-Service Package
- Complete the peanut ball proficiency skills checklist and other items in In-Service Training Package

WHERE DO I FIND AN AUTHORIZED PEANUT BALL TRAINER?

Our Authorized Peanut Ball Trainers have so much information to share and are great resources to follow. They also offer workshops, and can come on-site to train your staff or group. You will find all of our Authorized Trainers on the Premier Birth Tools website: premierbirthtools.com/authorized-peanut-ball-trainers

Cheri Grant

The Peanut Ball Lady

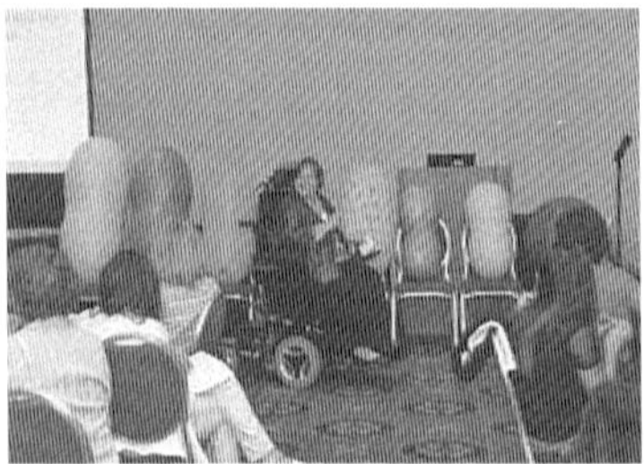

Location: Collinsville, Oklahoma
Email: Premierbirthtools@gmail.com

"Peanut Balls are one of the best tools to use in facilitating the birth of the baby to move through the pelvis."

Heather Turner

First Authorized Peanut Ball Trainer

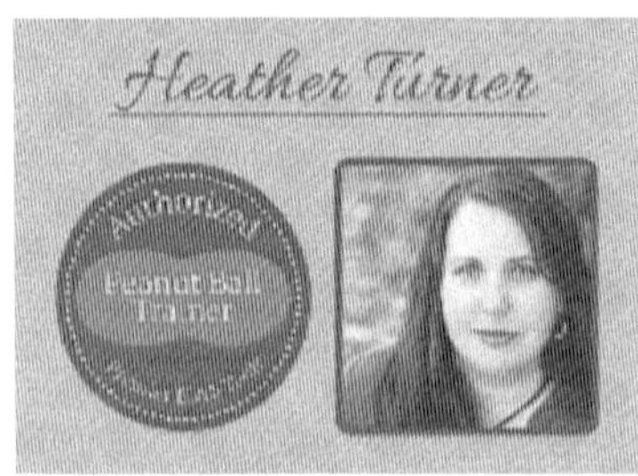

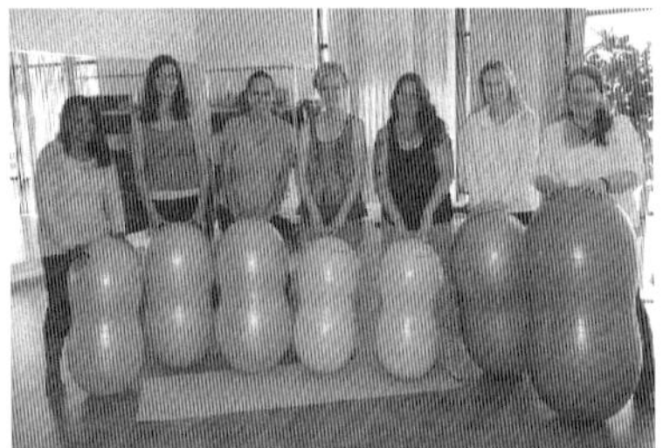

Location: Palmdale, California
Email: heather@navydoula.com
Resource(s): How-To Peanut Ball Workshop by Your Birth
Website: navydoula.com

"When I teach students, I draw their attention to how the Side-Lying Tuck Position opens the pelvis: 'Come over here and look at my bottom'."

Melissa Harley

Doula Trainer and Authorized Peanut Ball Trainer

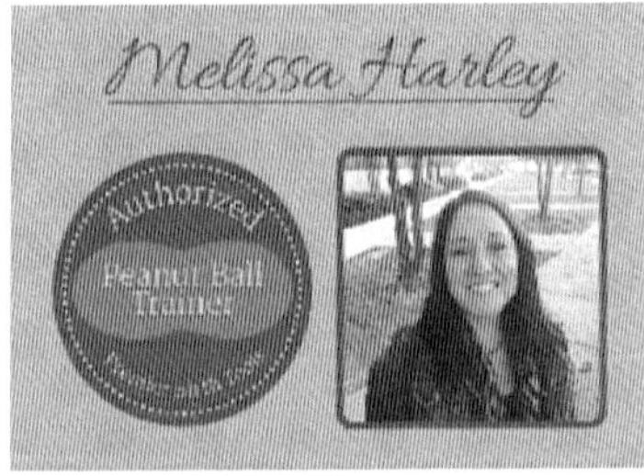

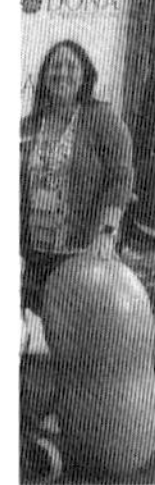

Location: Tallahassee, Florida
Email: capitalcitydoula@comcast.net
Resource(s): Doula Trainings by Capital City Doula Services, Techniques for Labor Progress Including Peanut Ball
Website: capitalcitydoulaservices.com

"Knowing the peanut ball is proven to shorten labors, using it is a wonderful addition to your bag of tools. Faster, more efficient labors? Yes please!"

Amy Brookwalter

Doula and Authorized Peanut Ball Trainer

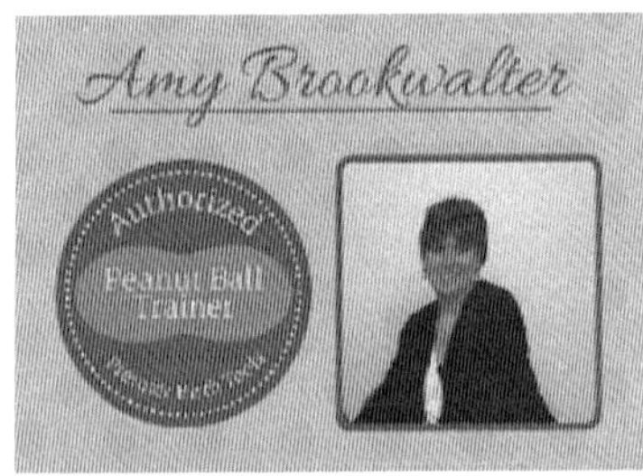

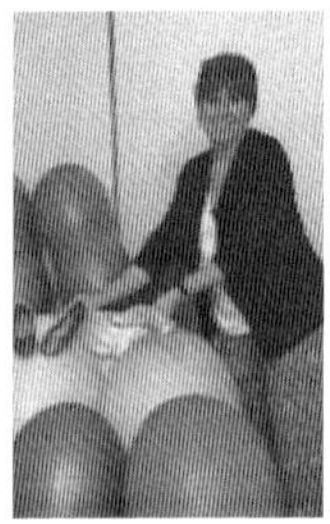

Location: Manassas, Virginia
Email: abookwalter@msn.com
Facebook: Rosebud Doula Services

"Remember to place feet where the baby is at pelvis: Top: Plié; Middle: Winshield Wipers; Bottom: Dorothy Kick."

Heidi Duncan

Authorized Peanut Ball Trainer

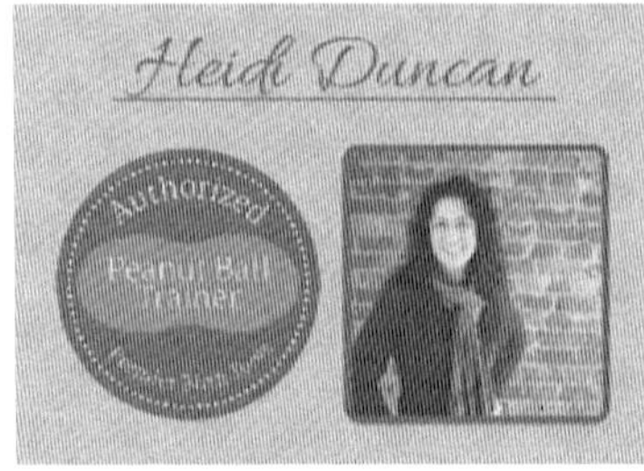

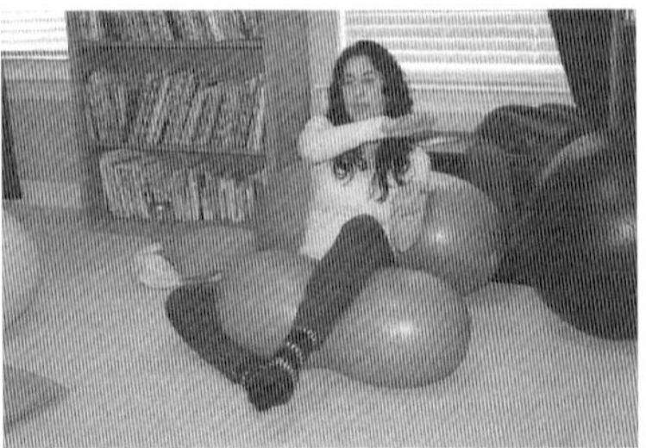

Location: Nashville, Tennessee
Email: expectingnewlifeteam@gmail.com
Resource(s): Peanut Ball Skills Workshops by Expecting New Life Birth Services
Website: expectingnewlife.com

"I don't know who the first person was to think of using a peanut ball for labor and birth support, but I'm grateful to them! It's such a versatile tool, yet with basic knowledge you can make a real difference in someone's labor experience. I'd say it's one of the best things to come into birth work in quite some time."

Amanda Irby

Nurse and Authorized Peanut Ball Trainer

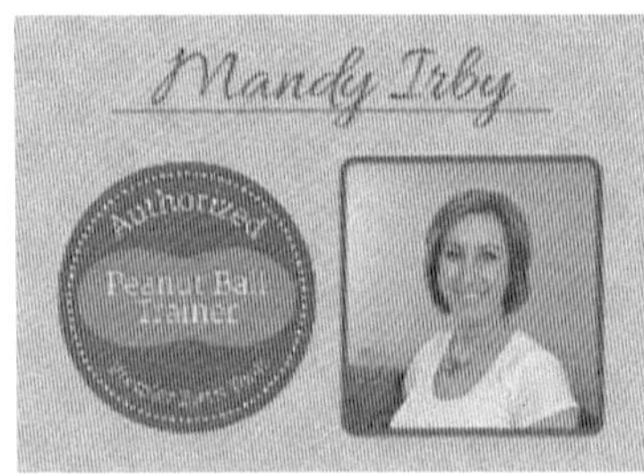

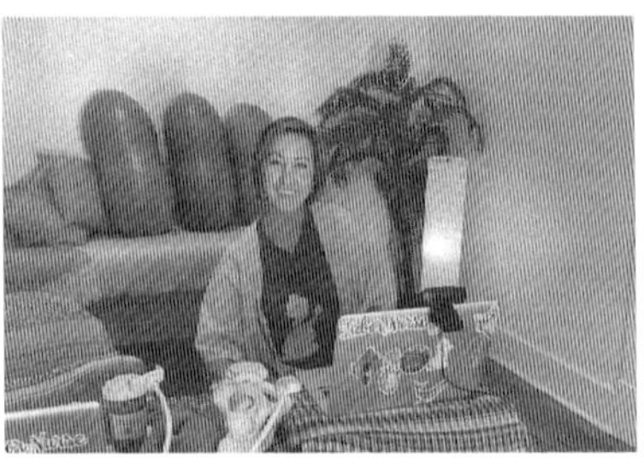

Location: Roanoke, Virgina
Email: Team@mandyirby.com
Resources: Workshops by The Birth Nurse™
Wesbite: Mandyirby.com/nurses

"Peanut balls are some of the most powerful tools in a L&D nurse's tool kit. They facilitate labor and trust at the same time!"

Amy Emerson

Nurse and Authorized Peanut Ball Trainer

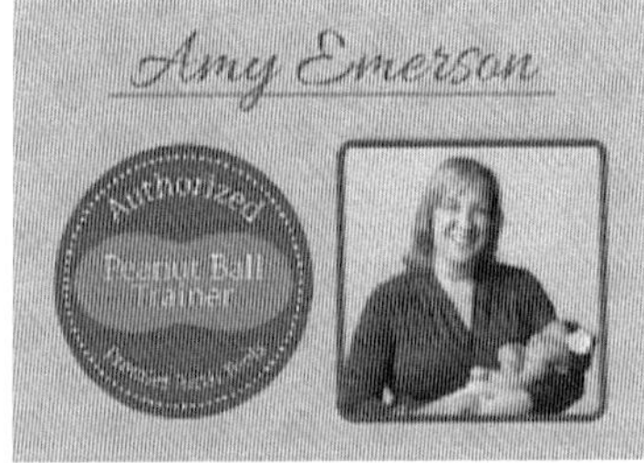

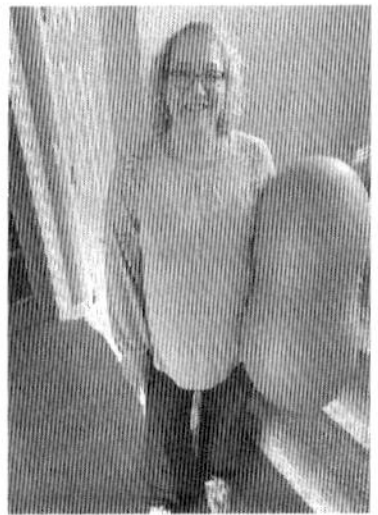

Location: Jenks, Oklahoma
Email: doulaforbirth@gmail.com

"Peanut balls help make room for the passenger, aka the baby. We're figuring out ways to make the pieces fit like in a puzzle. Baby has to come in, move through/down, and out!"

Emma Whitlock

Doula and Authorized Peanut Ball Trainer

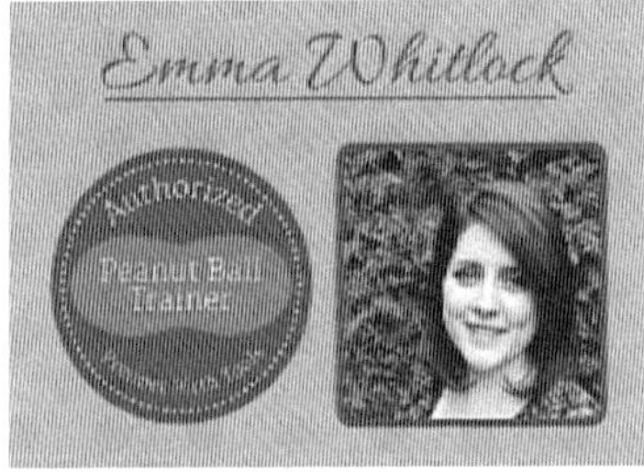

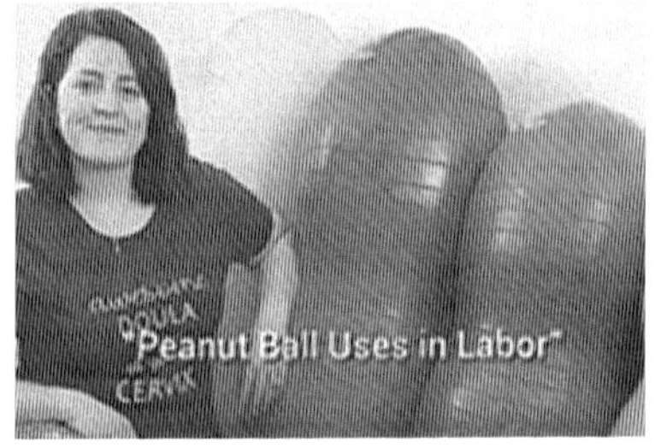

Location: Berea, Ohio
Email: thewombwithin@gmail.com

"What I like most about the peanut ball is how versatile it is for laboring at home and *in the hospital. So many people associate the peanut ball with keeping the hips open if there is an epidural placed, but I love being able to show families and providers all the different ways the peanut ball can be used for comfort, positions, pushing, resting, and so much more!"*

Marques Scott

Nurse and Authorized Peanut Ball Trainer

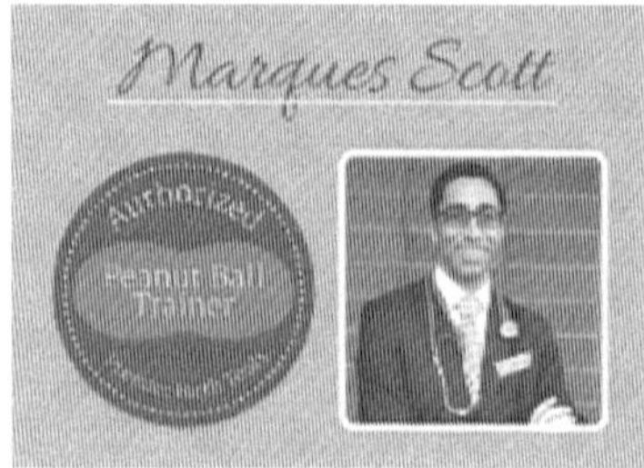

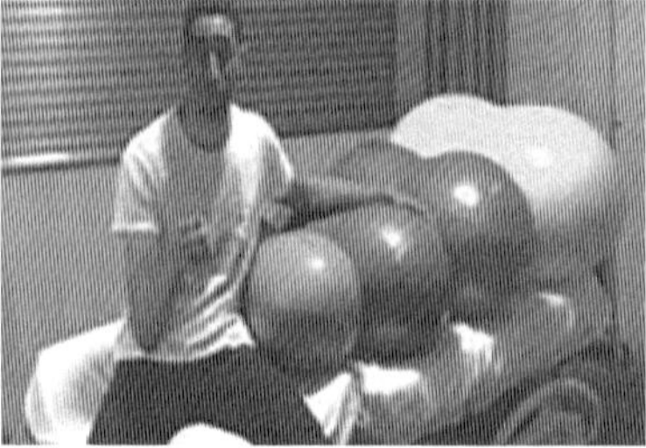

Location: Hillsboro, Oregon
Email: marques.scott@gmail.com

"I love teaching nurses how to use the peanut ball correctly."

Stephanie Assouline

Nurse and Authorized Peanut Ball Trainer

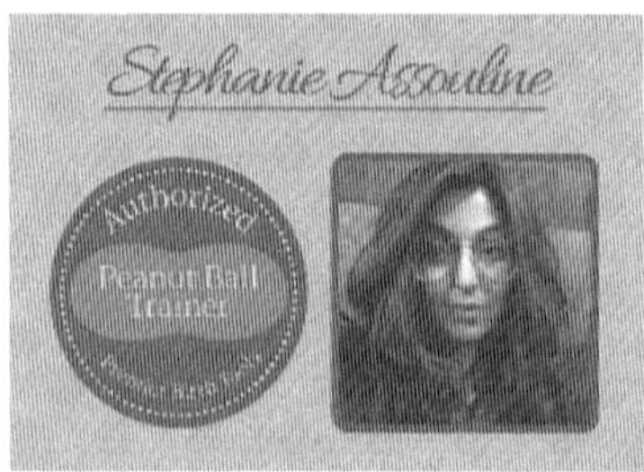

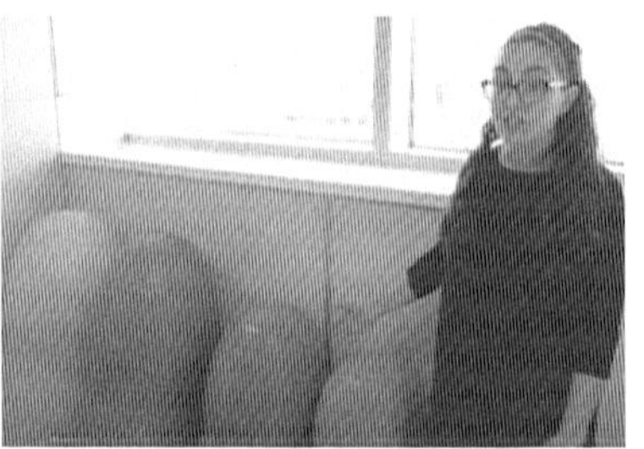

Location: Montreal, Quebec, Canada
Email: s.assouline.rn@gmail.com

"Don't underestimate the power of this peanut-shaped ball. I have witnessed it help many women with progressing their labors at surprising speed!"

Megan Honaker

Nurse and Authorized Peanut Ball Trainer

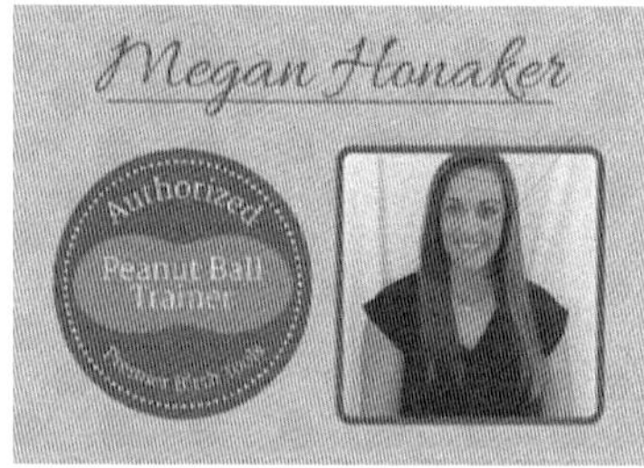

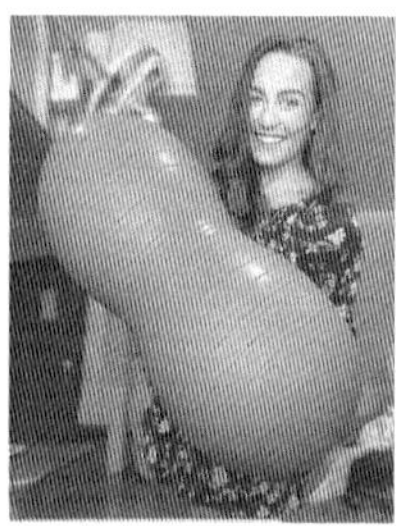

Location: Nashville, Tennessee
Email: megan.honaker@outlook.com

"The peanut ball is an easy-to-use, nurse-driven labor support tool! I love seeing nurses get excited to go 'peanut ball' their patients, knowing how beneficial this tool is in improving fetal rotation and maternal pelvic opening."

Nona Barnett

Nurse and Authorized Peanut Ball Trainer

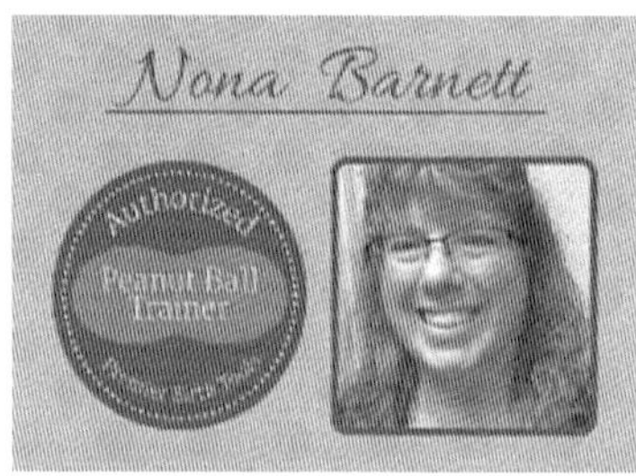

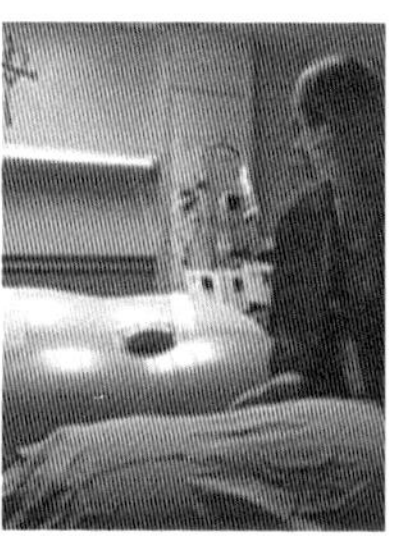

Location: Florence, Oregon
Email: barnett.nona@yahoo.com

"This peanut ball tool should be available for every delivery. It should be taught to every labor nurse—the same as teaching how to apply fetal monitoring devices."

Amy Wilt

Doula and Authorized Peanut Ball Trainer

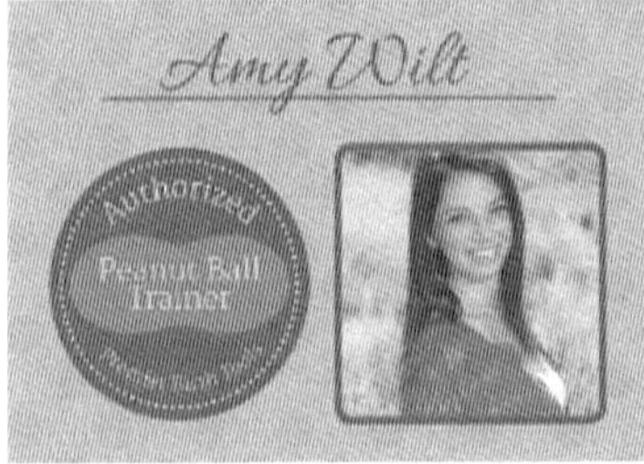

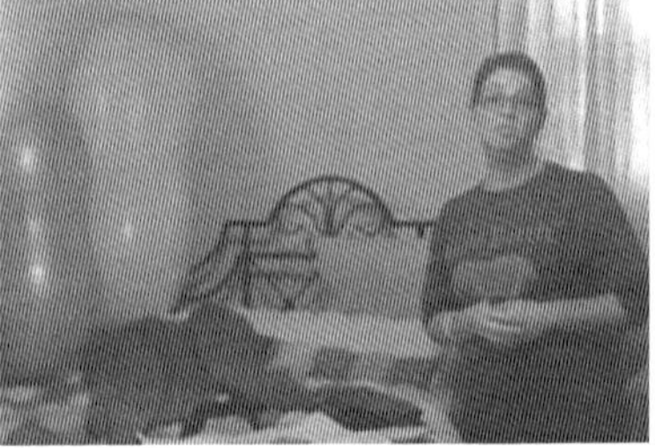

Location: Harrisburg, Pennsylvania
Email: amywiltdoula@gmail.com

"The peanut ball helps make labor and pushing way easier (and faster)! By using the ball to labor-down, it significantly reduces perineal tearing!"

As of this printing of this book, these are the Authorized Peanut Ball Trainers. For the most current list of Authorized Peanut Ball Trainers visit: premierbirthtools.com/authorized-peanut-ball-trainers

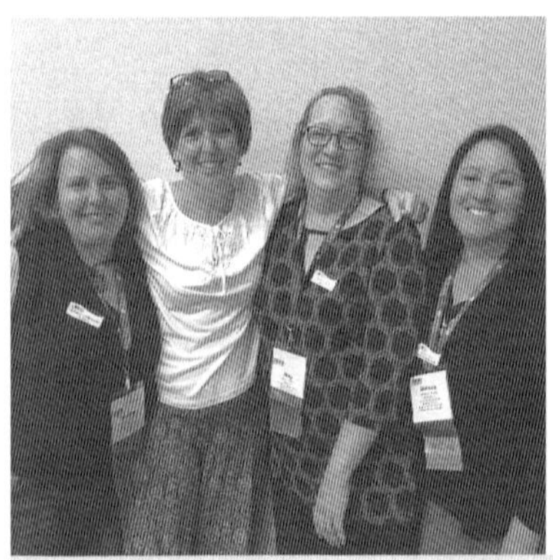

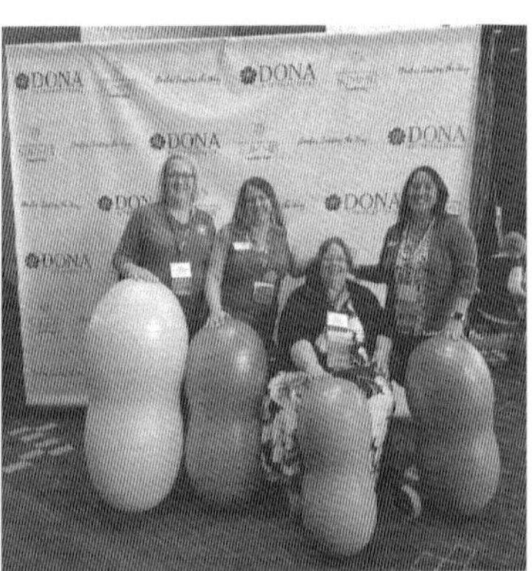

Authorized Peanut Ball Trainers at a convention.
Photo © courtesy Premier Birth Tools LLC

PEANUT BALL PACKET AND INFORMATION

- **FREE Premier Birth Tools Peanut Ball Informational Packet:** premierbirthtools.com/store/peanut-ball-doula-childbirth-educator-packet/
- **Set of 5 Peanut Ball Charts:** Includes 117 pictures, representing 65 different positions using the peanut ball. Premierbirthtools.com/store/peanut-ball-bundle-set-of-5-charts
- **Peanut Ball Training Packages:** Available as a physical package of material or as a download with everything you need. Premierbirthtools.com/store/peanut-ball-in-service-training-packages/
- **Peanut Ball Training Information:** premierbirthtools.com
- **Authorized Peanut Ball Trainers Workshops:** Visit Premier Birth Tools for more information. Some have in-person and others have virtual, online training.

Thanks so much! You guys are the best! It is so challenging, especially for birth moms right now. Thanks so much for all of the helpful pages of peanut ball positions!! These are all so helpful!

Donna B. Landeta, doula, Pennsylvania

WHERE CAN I FIND PEANUT BALL POSITIONS?

Premier Birth Tools website has the whole set of 5 peanut ball charts. These are laminated for easy cleaning and have pictures on both sides of the charts. They are 8x10 and easy to carry to a birth or to have in each labor room. Perfect with pcitures for demontrating which peanut ball postion you want to use next for a client in labor:
premierbirthtools.com/store/peanut-ball-bundle-set-of-5-charts

Peanut Ball Bundle, Set of 5 Charts

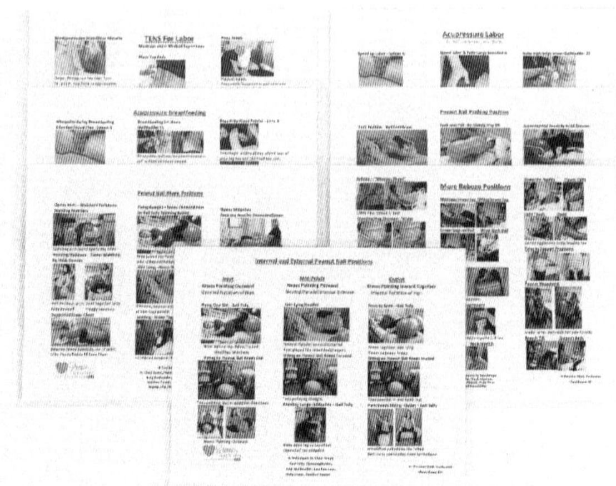

- Includes 117 pictures, representing 65 different positions using the peanut ball
- Peanut Ball Pushing Positions Chart
- Peanut Ball More Positions Chart
- Internal and& External Peanut Ball Positions Chart
- Original Peanut Ball Positions Chart
- New Peanut Ball Positions Chart
- These include labor, pushing, internal and external rotation of femurs, positions related to where the baby is in relation to pelvis, asymmetrical positions, opening the inlet, midpelvis, and outlet
- Also demonstrates positions with and without the epidural
- Illustrates all four sizes of peanut balls.
- Includes cleaning, covering, and choosing the correct size for your client

I am ordering more laminated charts! Yesterday I taught my DNP project. My director came to me and said that there are already requests to have this material in every labor room. The staff love them! Thank you for these charts. They are a wonderful product to help our nurses and patients.

Mimi Dent, labor and delivery nurse, CA

BIBLIOGRAPHY

"Ahmadpour, P, Mohammad-Alizadeh-Charandabi, S, Doosti, R, Mirghafourvand, M. Use of the Peanut Ball during Labour: A Systematic Review and Meta-Analysis. Nurs Open. 2021; 00: 1– 9. Https://Doi.org/10.1002/nop2.844." nurs open, 2021.

Alvarado, Yolanda, Lauren Outland, Angelica Menchaca, and Niki Strong. "Promoting the Progress of Labor With the Peanut Ball." Journal of Obstetric, Gynecologic & Neonatal Nursing 46, no. 3 (2017). https://doi.org/10.1016/j.jogn.2017.04.041.

Assouline, Stephanie. "***PEANUT BALL FOR LABOR (Basic+Advanced Positions) ***." YouTube video, 9:11, May 1, 2017. https://www.youtube.com/watch?v=WcE7wCNdTW0&t=145s.

Bell, Amy D., Saju Joy, Susan Gullo, Robert Higgins, and Eleanor Stevenson. "Implementing a Systematic Approach to Reduce Cesarean Birth Rates in Nulliparous Women." Obstetrics & Gynecology 130, no. 5 (2017): 1082–89. https://doi.org/10.1097/aog.0000000000002263.

Bell, Catherine. "Effectiveness of Using the Peanut Ball to shorten the first and Second Stage of labor" Nursing Education Research Conference 2018 https://sigma.nursingrepository.org/bitstream/handle/10755/623757/Bell_Info_89909.pdf;sequence=2

Baran, Gonca Karataş Baran 2021. "The Effect of Using a Birthing Ball (Peanut Ball) During Labor on the Labor Process" Ankara Yildirim Beyazıt University Study https://trialbulletin.com/lib/entry/ct-04729426

Blandine, Calais-Germain And Núria , Vives Parés, 2012. Preparing for a Gentle Birth: The Pelvis in Pregnancy. Healing Arts Press

Bookwalter, Amy. Peanut Ball Positions. Pictorial Home Birth Poster Presentation at 2017 DONA International Convention

Bueno-Lopez, Vanessa, Carmen Fuentelsaz-Gallego, Manel Casellas-Caro, Ana Maria Falgueras-Serrano, Silvia Crespo-Berros, Ana Maria Silvano-Cocinero, Carolina Alcaine-Guisado, Manuela Zamoro Fuentes, Elena Carreras, and Carmen Terré-Rull. "Efficiency of the Modified Sims Maternal Position in the Rotation of Persistent Occiput Posterior Position during Labor: A Randomized Clinical Trial." Birth 45, no. 4 (2018): 385–92. https://doi.org/10.1111/birt.12347.

Clutter, L. B.2016. "The Peanut Ball: A useful Tool for Labor & Delivery Support" 2016 Family Nursing International Conference

Clutter, L. B. & Grant, C. 2015. "Peanut Balls: Improving Options for Women Laboring with an Epidural." Australian Midwifery News, 15(3). 36-37

Craig, B., Grant, C. B., & Rice, A. 2014. "Length of labor reduced through use of peanut ball: A retrospective study". Unpublished manuscript.

Clutter, L. B.& Grant, C. B. 2014. "The Peanut Ball: A Remarkable Labor Support Tool. "International Doula, 22(4), 12-15.

Cockeram , Mindy 2020. "Narrow the Knees to Push with Ease: Challenge The Norm and Get The Job Done! "A Research Blog About Healthy Pregnancy, Birth & Beyond. Lamaze International. https://www.lamaze.org/Connecting-the-Dots/Post/narrow-the-knees-to-push-with-ease-challenge-the-norm-and160get-the-job-done-1

D'Angelo, R. & Harris, L. 2016. "Do peanut shaped birthing balls reduce the length of labor in patients with epidural analgesia?" ClinicalTrials.gov Identifier: NCT02539563. https://clinicaltrials.gov/ct2/show/NCT02539563?term=Peanut+Ball&rank=1

DeOliveira, Emily." EBP Poster Presentation: Can the use of peanut balls reduce the length of labor?" YouTube video, 5:53, March 26, 2016 https://www.youtube.com/watch?v=B3uYgLd77RE

Duncan, Heidi. "Peanut Ball Positions for Labor & Birth." YouTube video, 43:03, February 10, 2017. https://youtu.be/VlXOqs8q62g.

Evans, Sarah J., and Michelle M. Cremering. "Use of Peanut Labor Ball for Pelvic Positioning for Nulliparous Women Following Epidural Anesthesia." Journal of Obstetric, Gynecologic & Neonatal Nursing 45, no. 3 (2016). https://doi.org/10.1016/j.jogn.2016.03.119.

Ezuma, Ndidiamaka (2020) "The Use of the Peanut Ball on Nulliparous Women Laboring With An Epidural" Directed Scholarly Project, Bradley University. http://www.doctorsofnursingpractice.org/wp-content/uploads/project_form/complete_311220082949.pdf

Grenvik, Jessica M., Emily Rosenthal, Gabriele Saccone, Luigi Della Corte, Johanna Quist-Nelson, Richard D. Gerkin, Alexis C. Gimovsky, Mei Kwan, Rebecca Mercier, and Vincenzo Berghella. "Peanut Ball for Decreasing Length of Labor: A Systematic Review and Meta-Analysis of Randomized Controlled Trials." European Journal of Obstetrics & Gynecology and Reproductive Biology 242 (2019): 159–65. https://doi.org/10.1016/j.ejogrb.2019.09.018.

Grant, Cheri. 2021." Premier Birth Tools Peanut Ball Informational Nurse and Doula Packet." https://premierbirthtools.com/store/peanut-ball-nurse-packet/

Grant, Cheri. "How do Peanut Balls Support Labor? With Cheri Grant" Evidence Based Birth EBB 45 podcast, September 26, 2018, https://evidencebasedbirth.com/how-do-peanut-balls-support-labor/

Grant, Cheri. "The Peanut Ball and the Pelvis with Cheri Grant RN the "Peanut Ball Lady." Yoga Birth Babies podcast, September 16, 2019. https://prenatalyogacenter.com/blog/the-peanut-ball-and-the-pelvis-with-cheri-grant-the-peanut-ball-lady/

Heffernan, Conor. 2016." A brief history of the Swiss ball." https://physicalculturestudy.com/2017/12/27/a-brief-history-of-the-swiss-ball-2/

Hickey, Lisa, and Jane Savage. "Effect of Peanut Ball and Position Changes in Women Laboring With an Epidural." Nursing for Women's Health 23, no. 3 (2019): 245–52. https://doi.org/10.1016/j.nwh.2019.04.004.

Honaker, Megan Elizabeth, 2021 "The Use of a Peanut Ball During Labor in Nulliparous Term Singleton Vertex Pregnancies to Decrease the Primary Cesarean Rate: An Evidence-Based Practice Improvement Project" Graduate Publications and Other Selected Works - Doctor of Nursing Practice (DNP). Tennessee University https://trace.tennessee.edu/dnp/3

Honaker, Megan. "Using the Peanut Ball to Promote Vaginal Birth." YouTube video, 12:46, May 12, 2020, https://youtu.be/kP_IeKkfDzU

Irby, Mandy. "Shorten Labor | Faster Birth With Peanut Balls." YouTube video, 9:59. February, 25 2017. https://www.youtube.com/watch?v=B7m-FvB9-HsU

Irby, Mandy "What Does It Look Like to Push with Peanut Balls? // Peanut Balls in Labor." YouTube video, 17:59, March 13, 2019. https://www.youtube.com/watch?v=28NXJfQ8w1Y

Kwan, Mei, and Rebecca Mercier. "Impact of Peanut Ball Device on the Duration of Active Labor: A Randomized Control Trial." American Journal of Perinatology 35, no. 10 (2018): 1006–11. https://doi.org/10.1055/s-0038-1636531.

Klump, Jennifer S., (2017) "Use of the Peanut Ball to Reduce Cesarean Rate" (Publication No. 26) [Doctoral dissertation, University of Northern Colorado].https://digscholarship.unco.edu/capstones/26

Lee & Crawford (2018) "Peanut Ball Use by Women Labor: A review of Literature " http://kpscnursingresearch.org/wp- admin/images/Forms/Literative%20Evidence%20Summaries/Peanut%20Ball%20Literature%20Review_FINAL_April%202018.pdf

Logan, Linda, and Susan Stettler. "Reduction of Primary Cesarean Birth Rate in a Rural Hospital Driven By Nurse-Initiated Peanut Ball Use in Active Labor." Journal of Obstetric, Gynecologic & Neonatal Nursing 48, no. 3 (2019). https://doi.org/10.1016/j.jogn.2019.04.185.

Lythgoe, A. (2014). "Peanut Balls for Labor—A valuable tool for promoting progress? "A Research Blog About Healthy Pregnancy, Birth & Beyond. Lamaze International. Accessed July 25,2021 http://www.scienceandsensibility.org/?p=8166

Mackeen, Awathif D, Quinn. Shantel T 2019 "Geisinger Medical Center Reducing CesareanDelivery Rate in Obese Patients Using the Peanut Ball" https://clinicaltrials.gov/ct2/show/NCT03772886

Martinez-Rodriguez. A, Stairhime, C, "Use of Birthing Tools to Decrease Labor Times Houston Methodist Willowbrook " https://www.texaschildrens.org/sites/default/files/uploads/documents/health_professionals/kaleidoscope/Day%202%20Birthing%20Tools.pdf

MamasteFit Training. "Opening the Bottom of the Pelvis for Pushing (Outlet Opening)." YouTube, video, 1:17, December 24, 2019, https://www.youtube.com/watch?time_continue=1&v=sw8wR-2LRgo&feature=emb_logo

Milton, Sarah 2020 "Using the Peanut Exercise Ball to Reduce Cesarean Section Rates: A Randomized Controlled Trial" https://clinicaltrials.gov/ct2/show/NCT02899260

Outland, Lauren, and Yolanda Alvarado. "Preventing Cesareans with Peanut Ball Use." Journal of Nursing Education and Practice 10, no. 1 (2019): 107. https://doi.org/10.5430/jnep.v10n1p107.

Palladino, Jena, Erica R. Severi, Donna Bowman, and Elizabeth Kelley. "Nurse-Driven Labor Initiatives to Reduce Cesarean Rates." Journal of Obstetric, Gynecologic & Neonatal Nursing 48, no. 3 (2019). https://doi.org/10.1016/j.jogn.2019.04.048.

Payton, Carol L., 2015. "Use of the Peanut Ball to Decrease First and Second Stages of Labor." Graduate Theses, Dissertations, and Capstones, Paper 14. Bellarmine University http://scholarworks.bellarmine.edu/cgi/viewcontent.cgi?article=1013&context=tdc

Perez, Polly. 2000. Birth Balls: Use of Physical Therapy Balls in Maternity, Cutting Edge Press

Potter, Katherine, and Susan E. Brown Will. "Increasing Use of the Peanut Ball in Labor." Journal of Obstetric, Gynecologic & Neonatal Nursing 49, no. 6 (2020). https://doi.org/10.1016/j.jogn.2020.09.079.

Premier Birth Tools LLC. Peanut Ball Ambassador Application Interviews (2014-2021)

Roth, Cheryl, Sarah A. Dent, Sheryl E. Parfitt, Sandra L. Hering, and R. Curtis Bay. "Randomized Controlled Trial of Use of the Peanut Ball During Labor." MCN: The American Journal of Maternal/Child Nursing 41, no. 3 (2016): 140–46. https://doi.org/10.1097/nmc.0000000000000232.

Scott, Marques. "Labor with Peanut Balls," YouTube video, 9:12, April 1, 2017. https://youtu.be/qxTfKlCXqUI

Schmidt, M. & Roach, A. 2015. "A peanut and a pelvis: A simple change to facilitate labor and delivery." Science Internship Program: Nursing Care at Cleveland Clinic. http://civiceducation.clevelandclinic.org/getattachment/7cad7959-f19c-4f7b-b5a4-b7a4259ad476/A-Peanut-and-a-Pelvis-A-Simple-Change-to-Facilitat.aspx

Stulz, V., Campbell, D., Yin, B., Al Omari, W., Burr, R., Reilly, H., & Lawson, K. (2018). "Using a peanut ball during labor versus not using a peanut ball during labor for women using an epidural: study protocol for a randomized controlled pilot study." Pilot and Feasibility Studies, 4(1), 156. https://pilotfeasibilitystudies.biomedcentral.com/track/pdf/10.1186/s40814-018-0346-9

Simkin, Penny, Hanson, Lisa, And Ancheta, Ruth. 2017. The Labor Progress Handbook. (4th ed.) Malden, MA: Blackwell Science.

Smith H & Peterson N & Lagrew D & Main E. "Toolkit to support vaginal birth and reduce primary cesareans: a quality improvement toolkit." Stanford (CA) Maternal Quality Care Collaborative CMQCC- Updated 2018 with peanut ball section (2018) https://www.academia.edu/24991490/Toolkit_to_Support_Vaginal_Birth_and_Reduce_Primary_Cesareans_A_Quality_Improvement_

Spinning Babies ® "Three Levels of the Pelvis By: Gail Tully" Accessed July 25, 2021 https://www.spinningbabies.com/optimal-maternal-postions-at-the-levels-of-the-pelvis/

Tully, Gail. 2020. Changing Birth on Earth: A Midwife and Nurse's Guide to Using Physiology to Avoid Another Unnecessary Cesarean. Maternity House Publishing

Tussey, Christina Marie, Emily Botsios, Richard D. Gerkin, Lesly A. Kelly, Juana Gamez, and Jennifer Mensik. "Reducing Length of Labor and Cesarean Surgery Rate Using a Peanut Ball for Women Laboring With an Epidural." The Journal of Perinatal Education 24, no. 1 (2015): 16–24. https://doi.org/10.1891/1058-1243.24.1.16.

Tussey, Christina, and Emily Botsios. "Use of a Labor Ball to Decrease the Length of Labor in Patients Who Receive an Epidural." Journal of Obstetric, Gynecologic & Neonatal Nursing 40 (2011). https://doi.org/10.1111/j.1552-6909.2011.01243_25.x.

Turner, Heather. "Using the Peanut Ball by Your Birth." YouTube video, 8:34, April1,2015 https://www.youtube.com/playlist?list=PL5h-501qK0oo8FMy1UdWJZf_Dt9vqTIgAl

Whitlock, Emma. "Peanut Ball Uses in Labor." YouTube video, 7:38, March 22, 2018. https://www.youtube.com/watch?v=sOb2OJHGBwg

ABOUT THE AUTHOR

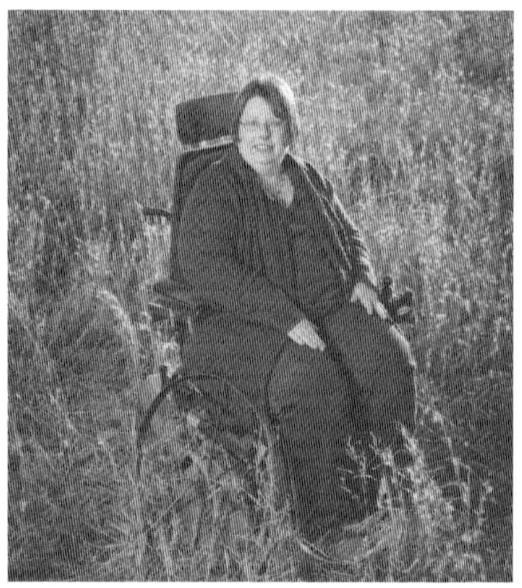

CHERI GRANT, RN, ICCE, CLC, ICBD, CLD, CD BDT(DONA) is known as "The Peanut Ball Lady" She is the coordinator of LifeStart Program at Ascension St. John Owasso Hospital. Childbirth Graphics named her "The Peanut Ball Lady." She is the founder and consultant for Premier Birth Tools, a website that has resources for peanut balls. Its mission is to get peanut balls in every hospital in the United States with resources for everyone in the world, and to teach how to use it correctly. She continues to guest lecture to residents and nurses on maternal and child health topics such as, the "Secrets of Labor Support." She spoke on the peanut ball at the National LAMAZE convention "The Peanut Ball: New Tool for Your Doula Bag and Its Effect on Laboring Women." She has also published several articles on the peanut ball, including "The Peanut Ball: A Remarkable Labor Support Tool" in the *DONA International Magazine* and the "Peanut Ball, Improving Options for Women Laboring with an Epidural" in *Australian Midwifery News*. She has recently been featured on the Podcast "How Do Peanut Balls Support Labor?" for Evidence Based Birth. She is an Authorized Peanut Ball Trainer and has developed many educational tools for the peanut ball. She also has given over 250 in-services on the peanut ball. She is the founder of Tulsa Doulas Inc. Doulas of Northeastern Oklahoma, which she started 29 years ago. She is a Birth DONA Doula Trainer; her certificate number is #2 as a trainer for DONA International. She has trained over 1,000 birth doulas. She is certified as a birth doula through DONA, ICEA, and CAPPA. She is an internationally certified childbirth educator through ICEA for over 30 years. Cheri is an author of "Labor Support Forms: A Guide to Doula Charting," which is in its third edition and on the app Mobile Doula. Several of her articles have been published in ICEA and DONA Journals. She has lectured at DONA International conventions, Gold Perinatal conference, and AWHONN State conventions "The Peanut Ball and Implications for Women Health." She also produced and directed a video on "Comfort Measures for Labor." She teaches and coordinates training workshops for birth doulas and nurses, talking about the profession of doulas around the country. She previously was a lactation consultant IBCLC for over 10 years. She also maintains her lactation educator. Previously she was also AWHONN certified in-patient obstetrical nurse for many years. She was also featured on the front page of the *Tulsa World* for her 42 years of work with pregnant and laboring women. She has now attended over 2,786 births in the last 50 years, working in Maternity and Labor and Delivery. She started before they allowed dads in the labor room. Today, she focuses on teaching and speaking about how to correctly use the peanut ball, which is her passion.

Thank you, Cheri, for sharing all your information about peanut balls!

Janet Elmeer, child birth educator, Indiana

Cheri waiting for Mia to be born. Bethany used many different peanut ball positions during her labor.

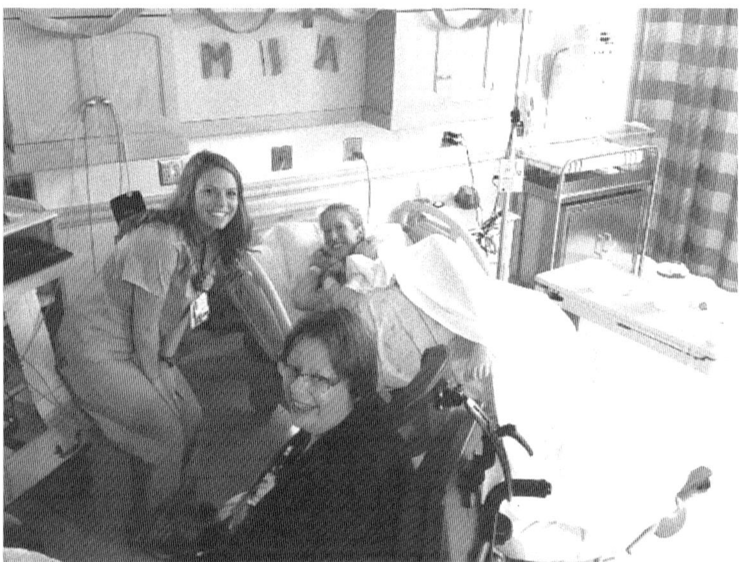

Bethany using Side-Lying Position on a peanut ball.

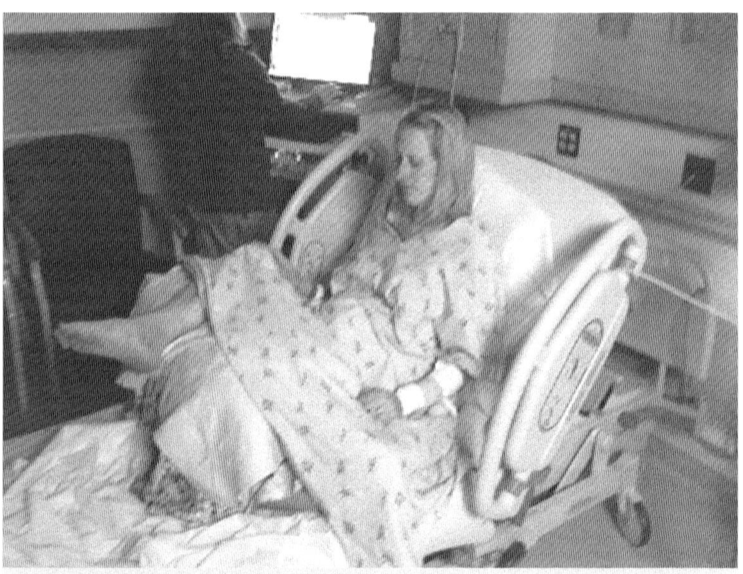

Bethany using Semi-Sitting Lunge on a peanut ball.

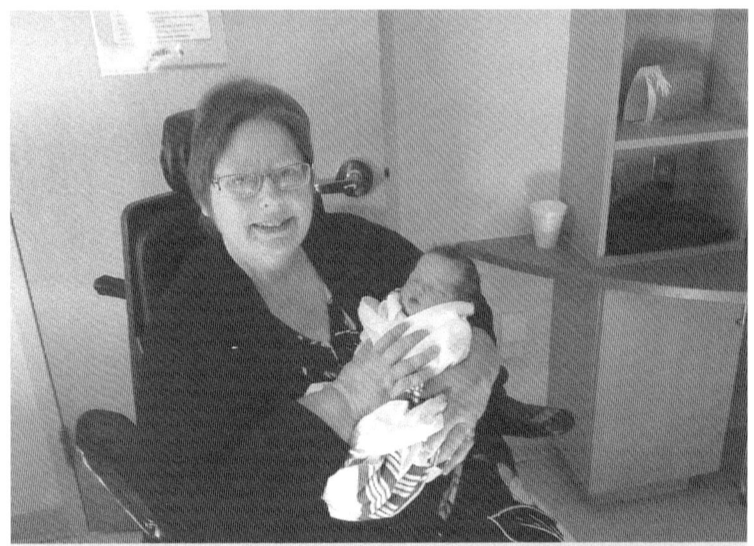

Cheri holding Mia. Cheri was Bethany's birth doula.

Photo © Premier Birth Tools LLC

The Peanut Ball is an Essential Labor Tool

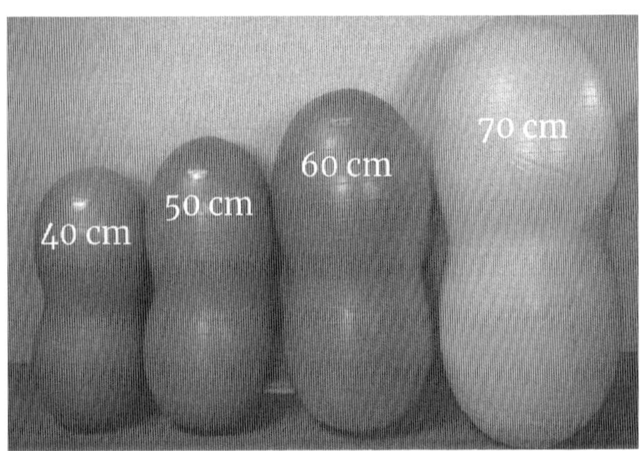

Give Birth With Balls 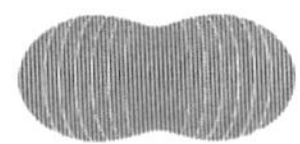

PREMIER BIRTH TOOLS, LLC

Cheri Grant, *RN, ICCE, CLC, ICBD, CLD, CD BDT(DONA) – Consultant*

Tiffany Graves – *Owner*

premierbirthtools.com

premierbirthtools@gmail.com

Find us on social media!

 @peanutballlady

 @PremierBirthTools

 @premier_birth_tools

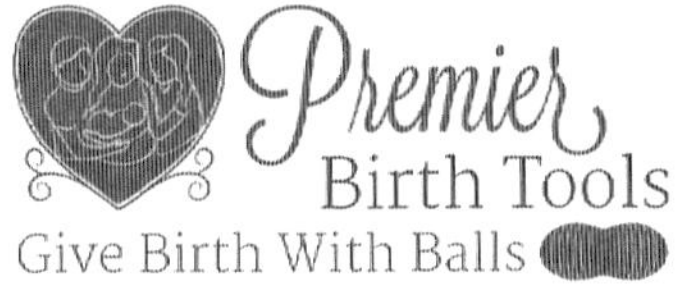

Visit PremierBirthTools.com for a FREE Peanut Ball Nurse Packet